A Sociological View of AIDS

This series, an academic masterpiece on AIDS research in the Chinese sociological community in the past two decades, analyzes in detail the situations of a range of people living with HIV/AIDS from various perspectives. By providing valuable theoretical insights and assessing counter measures, it not only allows readers to gain a thorough understanding of AIDS-related social realities, promotes the interpretation and implementation of social policies and the role of sociology in AIDS prevention and treatment, but also helps to coordinate the interests and needs of all party involved in order to handle relations between different groups of people and promote the formulation and adjustment of relevant policies, laws and regulations.

More information about this series at https://link.springer.com/bookseries/16458

Xiaoping Wang

Destigmatisation of People Living with HIV/AIDS in China

華中科技大學出版社
Huazhong University of Science and Technology Press

Springer

Xiaoping Wang
Shanxi Normal University
Taiyuan, China

Translated by
Zhiquan Zhang
Xinxiang Medical University
Henan, China

Leilei Liu
Xinxiang Medical University
Henan, China

Beijing Foreign Studies University
Beijing, China

ISSN 2662-5954 ISSN 2662-5962 (electronic)
A Sociological View of AIDS
ISBN 978-981-16-8533-0 ISBN 978-981-16-8534-7 (eBook)
https://doi.org/10.1007/978-981-16-8534-7

Jointly published with Huazhong University of Science and Technology Press
The print edition is not for sale in China (Mainland). Customers from China (Mainland) please order the print book from: Huazhong University of Science and Technology Press.

This Springer imprint is published by the registered company Springer Nature Singapore Pte Ltd.
The registered company address is: 152 Beach Road, #21-01/04 Gateway East, Singapore 189721, Singapore

Contents

Chapter 1
Introduction

> AIDS is not the most horrible thing. Worse comes to worst, that's death. The most horrible thing is losing your job. In addition, you will lose your companion. The society won't accept you. They want to isolate you. However, they can't kill you, but abandon you and let you die alone…
> —Quoted from one of the main characters of the Chinese movie *Tender Heart*

> The attitude towards people living with HIV/AIDS in China reflects the progress of civilisation in society. The stereotyped idea of 'talking about AIDS in a frightened attitude' must be discarded, and AIDS patients should be given more care.
> —Chinese Premier Li Keqiang

According to public reports, the AIDS epidemic is currently at a low prevalence level in China. However, there is a high prevalence in provinces such as Xinjiang, Sichuan, Yunnan, Guangxi, etc. The number of people living with HIV/AIDS (PLWHA) in the provinces of Yunnan, Guangxi and Sichuan accounts for 45% of the national cases in total. In 2014, the number of newly reported cases of PLWHA reached more than 10,000 in Sichuan, 9601 in Yunnan, and more than 5000 in Guangxi and Guangdong, respectively, with a sharp increase in the number of new infections in these regions in recent years. In terms of transmission routes, intravenous drug abuse and mother-to-child transmission have been reduced to the lowest level, while sexual transmission has become the main route. Among them, the increase in the transmission of men who have sex with men (MSM) is accelerating, and the proportion of elderly, middle-aged people and young students among PLWHA is increasing. Meanwhile, issues such as fear, discrimination and even insult rooted in society caused by AIDS have not been fundamentally solved; thus, the prevention and treatment of AIDS cannot be a "universal project". For instance, discrimination against PLWHA is widespread in terms of medical treatment, schooling, employment and consumption. For many families, PLWHA bring heavy mental and financial burdens to their family members or even bring catastrophes to their homes. Many people still regard AIDS as a "tiger" and have a fear of shaking hands with PLWHA, which virtually builds a "wall" between them so that PLWHA are discriminated against in daily life.

X. Wang, *Destigmatisation of People Living with HIV/AIDS in China*, A Sociological View of AIDS, https://doi.org/10.1007/978-981-16-8534-7_1

In view of the new development trend of AIDS and the results of epidemic surveillance, as well as the environment in which PLWHA live, it is necessary for the author to grasp, through in-depth interviews, the actual situation of AIDS transmission in China, the survival and social support status of PLWHA, as well as the psychology of PLWHA in discrimination and stigmatisation and the mechanisms at play, to provide references for the government and relevant departments in policy formulation.

1.1 Research Origin and Background

1.1.1 Research Origin

In 2004, I came into contact with the word "AIDS" from an event that happened on the train. A young mother with her 8-year-old child went to the Infectious Diseases Hospital of the city in which I worked to have a medical checkup for the child. At that time, she didn't tell me about the child's specific situation, and I didn't know that the child had been infected with AIDS. Coincidentally, we met on the train again. She narrated their sufferings, which shocked me greatly. The child, innocently infected because of blood transfusions, would experience hard times in his whole life. Another story is about one of my relatives. She was also infected through blood transfusion. After being diagnosed, she was discriminated against by her family members. She was helpless and behaved very cautiously. Initially, the word "AIDS" was strange to me, but now, people living with HIV/AIDS are around me.

Their stories and encounters have deeply motivated the author to help them. Moreover, the study of life-health issues from the sociological perspective rather than the public health perspective has always been the author's interest. It seems to the author that "life demands" on the basis of different understandings of life and health are one of the important driving forces of promoting social changes and progress. According to Hangsheng Zheng (2013), the important founder of Chinese sociology study and a professor of sociology at Renmin University of China, sociology studies the mechanism of social development and coordination development. Therefore, sociological research, which takes promoting the healthy development of society as its own responsibility, should make efforts to explore the constructive force of life demands and its mechanism of development. The elucidation of the social system changes at the macro level that requires a grand narration is beyond the author's reach. However, as a research beginner, the author deeply realises that the pursuit of the intrinsic value of human beings has typically been the driving force of social system changes in the process of in-depth research on specific social phenomena, such as the conceptual correctness of "women going astray". When endorsed and supported by a considerable number of individuals, certain value requirements have been disseminated through various forms (especially through the Internet with fast speed and great influence), which would demonstrate great power. In many cases, people are not clearly aware that their inner values (abstract subjective thoughts) reflect and identify the value pursuit in their inner hearts in the process of being confronted with reality and solving contradictions. It is undeniable that the pursuit of value is eventually implemented and achieved in the social movement.

If a social phenomenon can arouse discussions within a relatively wide range, it may constitute some kind of social issue and then further cause significant changes in thinking. Among the social issues involved in influential social phenomena, the impetus of values for change in social institutions often requires a micro-to-macro intermediary (usually in the form of a community or organisation) that enables the corresponding value pursuit to be realised in a planned, purposeful and organised way, thus constituting a tangible force that vigorously promotes changes (often more advanced and civilised) of the social system. It is within this conceptual framework that the book analyses the social phenomenon of AIDS in China, reveals how various stakeholders (PLWHA, ordinary people, etc.) act differently on the basis of different values and pursuits, and shows how the process provokes stigma and discrimination.

There are four main reasons for conducting the research. Firstly, sociologists should pay more attention to livelihood and vulnerable groups because human beings share a community of survival. Currently, AIDS is an incurable disease, and PLWHA are of lower social status and of awful survival situation. The discrimination caused by their terrible economic status and social status is worthy of attention and help. Secondly, the author has focused on the study of sociological theories for a long time. His research interests are the theory of stigma and its action mechanism, and the author has read a large number of relevant studies. The theory of stigma occurs to the author when choosing the study topic. Thirdly, the author participated in many AIDS forums and conferences and found that research on AIDS in China lacks sufficient data and literature. The available data and literature are mostly from the perspective of biology and medical physiology. However, there are relatively few studies from the perspectives of sociology, anthropology, social policy and social security, so the author devotes more attention to sociological research on AIDS, which systematically examines the relevant literature on sociology research of AIDS and builds up systematical theories, providing material support for future sociological research and national policy. Fourth, domestic research on PLWHA is mainly directed at people who are infected through blood transfusions, and there are few studies on people infected through sexually transmitted routes on female or male sex workers. Thus, the author resolutely decides to devote to the stigma study of AIDS, enlarging the scope of the research object and presenting the real situation of marginalised people.

1.1.2 Research Background

1.1.2.1 Status Quo of AIDS Transmission

Since the first case of AIDS was discovered in 1985, it has been reported that there are a total of 575,000 cases of PLWHA alive and 154,000 deaths up to October

2015. The day before World AIDS Day in 2014, Dr. Bernhard Schwartländer, WHO Representative in China, argued that one of the major challenges for China is that the HIV infection rate among men who have sex with men (MSM) is increasing and among heterosexual people is not decreasing. However, the HIV infection rate among injecting drug abusers has fallen significantly.

By the end of October 2015, PLWHA in China accounted for 0.06% of the total population of the country. It is worth noting that 97,000 new cases were recorded from January to October 2015, of which heterosexual transmission accounted for 66.6% and male-to-male transmission reached 27.2%. The proportion of male-to-male transmission rises significantly, with the average monthly infection rate reaching 8% in the last ten months.

AIDS not only significantly influences infected individuals and their families, but is also closely linked to a country's demographic structure, social stability, economic development and national prosperity.

Firstly, AIDS is directly related to numerous demographic issues, such as population size, national quality and structure, as well as health, welfare and security. For example, population loss will change the age structure, increase the ageing index, accelerate the ageing of the country and reduce the life expectancy per capita.

Secondly, AIDS indirectly affects the speed and quality of a country's economic development. Chinese scholars such as Liu et al. (2003) apply the economic growth model to systematically analyse the impact of AIDS on individuals, families and the economy and estimate that the cumulative impact of AIDS on the country's economy reached 300 million to 700 million yuan. Li et al. (2007) qualitatively analyse the economic relationship between AIDS and individuals, households, production sectors, health care sectors, regional economic trade and financial situation, and they estimate that the total loss of human capital due to AIDS in China in 2006–2010 would reach 200 million yuan.

Thirdly, AIDS is a threat to social harmony, stability and security. PLWHA are afflicted with social exclusion and discrimination in China and beyond, and they have no access to equal employment and medical treatment. All of these factors make people with suspected infection reluctant to undergo medical tests and make them conceal their real condition even if found to be positive, thereby increasing the risks of HIV transmission to some extent. Some HIV-infected people feel desperate and socially abandoned after being discriminated against, thus resorting to irrational behaviour for retaliation.

Currently, AIDS is a global concern because of its harmful effects. Although our government is highly concerned about the status quo and the development trend of the AIDS epidemic and has stepped up prevention and control efforts through various systems and means (with greater government efforts in medical care), individuals have been neglected. Although the laws, policies and services for PLWHA are improving, they, implemented at the macro level, ignore the individual differences and real needs of PLWHA. As a result, the services provided by the government and society do not truly meet their needs. For example, PLWHA, extremely sensitive under the double pressure of life crisis and public opinion, are more concerned about whether their personality is respected and their emotions are satisfied. If they are ignored, self-denial or even misanthropy may be evoked, making it difficult for them to adapt to society. Therefore, we should focus on their individual differences, highlight their emotional needs and psychological changes, and provide constructive suggestions and recommendations based on a full understanding of the inner crisis they face in their lives.

AIDS was once considered "plague" because there were no drugs to control the spread of the virus, resulting in a rapid onset and a few months of survival after diagnosis. By the mid-1990s, with advances in medicine, AIDS had gone from a terminal illness to a chronic illness, with the average number of infected persons living more than seven years. The longer life span has led to the realisation that PLWHA can no longer run away from the disease and deny its existence but need to "live with it" (which is still not so easy today).

Bury contends that "illness, and especially chronic illness, is precisely that kind of experience where the structures of everyday life and the forms of knowledge which underpin them are disrupted. Chronic illness involves recognition of the worlds of pain and suffering, possibly even of death" (1982: 169). Influenced by Giddens's term "critical situations" (1984: 61), Bury points out that chronic illness greatly disrupts the patient's life course and, most importantly, one's life experiences accumulated over many years (including role adaptation and coping) and had a profound impact on one's identity, which would cause the individual's existing values to be contradictory and be in a crisis (because the individual's self-values are related to the previous social identity, and it's difficult for patients to play the two conflicting identities). Chronic illnesses not only bring physical suffering but also make patients question their personal identity and individual values. PLWHA may have the following questions: "I know who I used to be, but who am I now?", "Where do I belong?" and "How to live in society?" The questions bring forth a crisis of identity. For them, the demonisation and stigmatisation of their identity causes them to suffer from the interplay of conflicting forces of self and social resistance as they adjust to this new identity and role, and identify with the new group to which they belong. Denial of their patient status leads to endless confusion and anxiety, while passive acceptance leads to low self-esteem and anxiety. Thus, the new identity not only affects their emotional and internal experience, but also hinders the successful completion of self-care behaviours and the achievement of self-management.

1.1.2.2 Status Quo of HIV Stigma

Firstly, PLWHA are afraid of being stigmatised in various ways, so they conceal their infection and continue to engage in unsafe behaviours (such as condomless sex and sharing needles), which in turn lead to the spread of HIV. Secondly, stigma has become a major stumbling block to timely testing, treatment and prevention of HIV, as high-risk groups (such as "female sex workers") are reluctant to get tested for fear of social sanctions, making it impossible to effectively control the spread of HIV. Worse still, PLWHA experience social stigma, discrimination, rejection and isolation, resulting in low self-esteem, low self-efficacy, depression, anxiety, despair and other negative psychological states, which in turn lead to excessive psychological stress. Living under such psychological pressure for a long time will lead to an unbalanced mentality and may resort to extreme methods (e.g., casual sex, etc.) to spread HIV, expecting others to contract HIV to take revenge on society, which will, in turn, jeopardise social stability and unity. HIV stigma is not only unhelpful to the "prevention of HIV" but has become a major "accomplice" in the spread of HIV. Therefore, by describing and analysing the status quo of stigmatisation of PLWHA and suggesting targeted and effective strategies, it will help to slow down the spread of HIV, alleviate their psychological and survival stress, and provide a harmonious social environment for this group.

1.1.2.3 Status Quo of Research on AIDS in China

In the mid to late 1980s, the social problems caused by AIDS aroused extensive and in-depth research in the academia of Europe and America. In social science research, scholars launched a series of studies on AIDS from the perspectives of labelling theory, social identity theory, feminism and queer theory. As the medical science community has not yet developed effective drugs to prevent and treat AIDS, "behavioural interventions" are considered to be an effective means, and the approach is directly related to different theories, such as cognitive theory, information diffusion theory, and subculture theory. In addition, theories such as globalisation and justice theory are relevant to the study of AIDS. In short, the study of AIDS has taken on a certain scale and has been described as the sociology of AIDS. Currently, epidemiology continues to dominate the discourse of AIDS research, while the social sciences have begun to shift their perspective from ethics to sociology.

1.2 Research Objects and Specific Issues

1.2.1 Research Objects

The book studies the stigmatisation of PLWHA, such medical terms as AIDS, HIV, and PLWHA, as well as the sociological concept of stigma and the causes, specific manifestations and social mechanisms of the social phenomenon.

The stigma of AIDS is generated by the differential treatment of PLWHA by the public, such as the negative attitudes, including negative stereotypes, emotional reactions and discriminatory behaviour, of non-infected people towards PLWHA, which hinders the treatment of AIDS.

AIDS stigma has been popular since the discovery of HIV, and the study of AIDS stigma has become a hot topic in academia. Currently, there are several major definitions of the concept of AIDS stigma.

Firstly, early researchers defined AIDS stigma as discrimination. The long incubation period of HIV and the incurable nature of AIDS itself have led to social discrimination against PLWHA and have seriously disrupted their daily life, and the discrimination against them is AIDS stigma. This definition simply equates AIDS stigma with behavioural discrimination, ignoring the cognitive and emotional components of stigma.

Secondly, AIDS stigma was regarded as a social process of aggravating social inequality and a form of social control (e.g., through moral critique, controlling the behaviour of PLWHA). Deacon (1994) argues that AIDS stigma is a process of change and confrontation (related to social change) between PLWHA and the society in which they live (social norms vary from country to country).

Thirdly, AIDS stigma was regarded as an emotional response. Joffe (1999) emphasises that the stigma of AIDS is an instinctive response to the risk of infection (e.g., the instinct to protect one's life) and that when individuals are exposed to a threatening situation (e.g., HIV infection), they denounce the stigmatised group and control the risk through social isolation, thus ensuring that they would not become infected and they are in a safe social environment.

The last one is that AIDS stigma was regarded as an attitude. Numerous researchers have applied different research methods to explore stigma against AIDS in three dimensions: cognitive, affective and behavioural aspects, including aspects of public stereotypes, attitudes and discriminatory behaviour towards the stigmatised individual or group. According to Goffman, negative public attitudes towards PLWHA generated HIV stigma.

1.2.2 Specific Issues

This study examines the dynamic process of the construction of the social identity of PLWHA and explores the laws of the social construction and self-construction of their identity, specifically addressing the following questions.

Along with the pathological change from the general population to the physical body of PLWHA, how is the stigmatising identity of PLWHA imposed and given to this group by society as a whole? What forces play an important role in the process?

How do PLWHA break through the stigma imposed by external structures and reshape their own identities in the face of the constant destruction of their existing lives and cognitive systems? What logic of action and values are implicit in these actions?

What kind of identity do PLWHA eventually acquire? What are the cultural and social constructions involved in this identity? In the process of identity reconstruction, how do the forces of structure and action play out and interact with each other? What are the main mechanisms of identity construction for this marginalised group?

These are the key questions that the researchers have to address.

1.3 Significance of the Study

Among the public health issues that have come to the fore since the first case of AIDS, AIDS has been the subject of scrutiny from the public, academia and policy makers. Not only has it been the most serious public health event since the 1980s, but it is also a growing social and even political issue of worldwide concern and has become the first controversial issue to be revisited by the world from social, cultural, economic, political and human rights perspectives.

1.3.1 Theoretical Significance

Studies on external and implicit attitudes towards AIDS stigma represent different psychological processes and mechanisms (such as behavioural and psychological rejection). Most current research on AIDS stigma relies on questionnaires and interviews to obtain external, superficial descriptive information but hardly touches on the internal, deep-seated mechanisms, especially the relationship between implicit and explicit attitudes of stigmatised groups, and does not produce a relatively unified view. In this regard, a systematic study of the social mechanisms of HIV stigma, especially the transmission modes, the role of the media, the extent of stigmatisation and the specific impact on PLWHA, and the search for specific sociological theories to explain the principles of stigmatisation, will provide a new research perspective for HIV stigma research.

Although China is now entering a period of rapid spread of the AIDS epidemic, there are few sociological studies on the relationship between the disease and stigma, especially from the perspective of PLWHA. Among the current studies on AIDS in China, some literature, to reduce AIDS discrimination, has mostly addressed the issue of AIDS discrimination from the perspective of medical ethics in terms of upholding human rights (advocating that PLWHA should enjoy the same rights as the general public), reducing discrimination, playing the role of the media, and publicising AIDS knowledge.

According to the researcher Ruotao Wang of the Chinese Centre for Disease Control and Prevention (China CDC), AIDS-related discrimination is non-institutional, but a socio-cultural discrimination that is not specifically directed at PLWHA, and the solution is a comprehensive transformation of social and cultural norms rather than just institutional reform. There are three major moves towards cultural change: resistance comes first, where vulnerable groups defend their rights; the second is universal education, advocating human rights, the rule of law, respect for the human personality and equality for all; and the third is social movements, which promote ideological enlightenment campaigns through media involvement in individual cases.

In sum, these studies fall far short of adequately explaining the socio-cultural context of AIDS stigma and exclusion, whether from a theoretical research perspective or from a practical research perspective on reducing discrimination, and fail to clearly articulate the multiple operational mechanisms and deep symbolic meanings of AIDS stigma.

1.3.2 Significance for Policy-Making

The stigmatisation of PLWHA has led some of them to deliberately conceal their condition, not daring to show their true identity, thus delaying detection and treatment of HIV, increasing the probability of infection due to contact with PLWHA, and augmenting the likelihood of transmission and the risk factor for HIV threatening society. Professor Dun Li of Tsinghua University points out from the different institutional backgrounds of the Chinese mainland and other countries and regions that AIDS discrimination in the Chinese mainland is mainly manifested as institutional discrimination. In today's world of establishing people-centred and life-respecting values, we should have a cognition and decision-making capacity and take anti-discrimination actions at the institutional level. Therefore, a comprehensive study of the current situation and specific process of stigmatisation of PLWHA and a full understanding of the mechanisms and principles of stigmatisation will help the government and health departments introduce reasonable and effective policies and regulations on HIV testing, which will have great significance for government departments to obtain real data on PLWHA and facilitate scientific formation and formulation of policies, thereby promoting AIDS-related research and the protection of basic rights of PLWHA.

1.3.3 Realistic Significance

The research results on the stigmatisation of PLWHA, if adopted by government departments, health departments, schools and other relevant institutions, will help to alleviate people's fear towards PLWHA, eliminate misunderstanding and prejudice, promote the construction of a friendly social environment for PLWHA, improve their living conditions, increase their well-being, and help them restore a secure and non-discriminatory life, which is of great significance.

Although AIDS is caused by the virus, it is indirectly transmitted by fear, rejection and prejudice. The public holds negative attitudes towards PLWHA, which, to some extent, hinders AIDS treatment. Stigma towards PLWHA makes it difficult to intervene, prevent and treat HIV and has a detrimental effect on their lives. Therefore, it is important to explore the status quo of HIV stigma and its mechanisms, analyse the influencing factors, and find ways to effectively intervene in HIV stigma to help reduce the psychological pressure on PLWHA, effectively control the spread of HIV, and successfully carry out HIV prevention and treatment.

Social discrimination and exclusion render stigmatised PLWHA in great physical suffering as well as enduring psychological and emotional upset, so their need and expectation for emotional support will be stronger, and if their expectation is not fulfilled, it will arouse fear, anxiety, anger, sadness, desperateness, etc. Additionally, they will also face anxiety in terms of broken families, loss of jobs, loss of financial resources, etc. These factors will bring them trauma and make it difficult to adapt themselves to society, which is not conducive to social harmony and stability. Therefore, the study aims to apply emotion theory to study the emotions of PLWHA, to provide them with emotional support and to enable them to take initiatives and to regulate emotions. The resolution of these issues is of great practical importance to the improvement of the quality of life and the survival environment of AIDS community, as well as the sound development of society as a whole.

1.4 Theoretical Originality and Issues to Be Explored

1.4.1 Originality in Research

The originality of the study is to apply social exclusion theory, welfare pluralism theory, actor theory and stigma theory to the socio-cultural mechanisms of stigmatisation of PLWHA.

Firstly, the scope of the research group has been broadened. It covers not only the group of infections through blood transfusion but also paid blood donors, men who have sex with men (MSM) and female sex workers. The study focuses on stigma, quality of survival and social support of the three groups. Through comparison, the study explores their common dilemmas and problems, focusing on the current situation and psychological mechanisms of social stigmatisation of the three groups.

Secondly, the impact of HIV stigma on the quality of survival is also studied. Through in-depth interviews, the study examines the influence of various factors of social support on the quality of survival, explains the intensity of stigma and the quality and satisfaction of government support, and proposes specific countermeasures to improve the quality of survival of PLWHA.

1.4.2 Issues to Be Explored

Attribution theory is often accepted by researchers as a mechanism for the formation of stigma; however, the theory does not explain stigma of various kinds. It has to do with complex causes of AIDS stigma, involving the institutions of a society and traditional culture of the nation. In recent years, some researchers have advocated the study of stigma from social and cultural perspectives, which suggests that AIDS stigma in different cultural contexts should be explored through cross-cultural research to verify the mechanisms of social and cultural processes that contribute to the production of AIDS stigma. Therefore, it will be an important perspective for future research to improve and develop attribution theory, explore the mechanisms of stigmatisation from social and cultural perspectives and formulate corresponding interventions.

In addition, most of the early AIDS studies used qualitative interviews with PLWHA or the general public to examine their attitudes and concerns. In recent years, following the UNAIDS (Joint United Nations Programme on HIV/AIDS) proposal to optimise questionnaires on AIDS stigma, a number of studies have emerged that validate measurement tools and investigate the attitudes of PLWHA or the general population through questionnaires. However, the generalisation of the findings obtained from both the interviews and questionnaires has been somewhat limited by the absence of a control group, which makes it difficult to conduct comparative studies and is subject to being questioned. In future studies, there is a great need to add experimental designs or to combine some experiments in survey studies to address the difficulties, and there should be long-term research considerations.

References

Bury M (1982) Chronic illness as biographical disruption. Sociol Health Illn 4(2):167–182

Deacon HJ (1994) A history of the medical institution on Robben Island, Cape Colony, 1846–1910. PhD thesis, University of Cambridge. https://doi.org/10.17863/CAM.19401

Giddens A (1984) The constitution of society: outline of the theory of structuration. Polity Press

Joffe H (1999) Risk and "the other." Cambridge University Press

Li J, Ren H (2007) The impact of AIDS on China's economy and society in 2006–2010. Academics 02:49–59

Liu K, Yuan J (2003) The AIDS epidemic and the impact on China's society and economy. Xuehai 05:68–72

Zheng H (2013) Introduction to sociology (A new revision). People's University of China Press

Chapter 2
Theoretical Foundations of Research on Stigmatisation of People Living with HIV/AIDS

2.1 Construction and Characteristics of Stigmatisation of People Living with HIV/AIDS

Any social phenomenon is the result of the mutual construction of individuals, individuals and society in a particular social environment. The process of interpreting and problem-solving any social phenomenon is also a process of mutual construction. The study of AIDS stigma must also be approached from a constructivist perspective.

2.1.1 Research on the Construction of Stigmatisation of People Living with HIV/AIDS

Social construction theory is the dominant theory in the study on AIDS from gender perspectives and behaviour change. Among the fifteen articles focusing on AIDS and construction, available on the journal website, most explore the construction of AIDS by the mass media from the perspective of media coverage, while some examine the definition of the concept of AIDS from the perspective of construction theory, and some examine construction theory.

Zhang et al. (2014) hold that the concept of AIDS has not only connoted medical knowledge but also connoted moral judgments. They argue that both scientific and ethical connotation have been defined by scientists holding different values, interest groups, political and social groups, and the mass media. Therefore, the concept of AIDS, believed to originate from socio-cultural construction, is coined under the impact of economic interests, political demands, value orientations and power relations and is a consensus in social interaction, in which the media plays an important role. These non-medical factors, such as political considerations, economic conditions, cultural characteristics, behavioural habits, organisational structures, and group

X. Wang, *Destigmatisation of People Living with HIV/AIDS in China*, A Sociological View of AIDS, https://doi.org/10.1007/978-981-16-8534-7_2

identity, transform AIDS from a medical issue to a social one, thereby making the socio-cultural discussion one of the important components of the conceptual system of AIDS.

Chen (2012) investigates the role of the media in the study of AIDS issues through an empirical approach. Dr. Chen argues that the media, as an important way for the public to obtain information about AIDS in modern society, undoubtedly functions importantly in the dissemination of HIV/AIDS knowledge and plays an irreplaceable role in the formation and change of public attitudes towards AIDS.

Dr. Chen's thesis focuses on the following issues. Firstly, the study presents the media's construction of AIDS issues in terms of data and, on this basis, focuses on the means by which the media constructs the attributive agenda of AIDS issues. The study finds that there is no direct relationship between the media's construction of AIDS issues and the real world. Different forms of media, such as various types of newspapers, vary in terms of circulation area, attributes and rank but do not show significant differences in the topics, genres, sources, layout of the stories, word choice or tone of the stories. The fact is that the newspapers also show a high degree of similarity in their media agendas on AIDS issues.

Secondly, Dr. Chen's study incorporates a detailed analysis of the public agenda as well as the policy agenda of the AIDS issue in the analysis of the specific agenda-setting process. It points out that policy agendas play a driving role in the agenda-setting process and function directly and noticeably in the agenda-setting of media. One evident conclusion is that policy agendas directly affect the setting and final positioning of AIDS issues and have an immediate impact on the phasing of media coverage of AIDS, while policy agendas also significantly influence the public agenda. It is important to note that there are significant differences between Western and Chinese society in these respects. For example, the media agenda is usually more active in Western society, but in Chinese society, the public is more passive on AIDS issues; that is, the public reacts passively to the construction of most relevant issues and is overwhelmingly submissive to the policy agenda. It is known that the public agenda is the ultimate target of both media agenda and policy agenda, but in fact, it is not given sufficient attention, and the reverse influence of public agenda on the other agendas is rather weak.

According to Dr. Chen, the present researchers generally agree that the media's construction of the AIDS issue has developed to a more scientific and humane stage since 2003. However, it cannot be denied that, in a particular social context, the development of the media is profoundly influenced by external factors such as political, economic and cultural aspects, by its own organisational goals and the interaction between media organisations, and by the framework of news production and the personal qualities of journalists. Consequently, there are still some problems in the construction process of the media about the AIDS issue. For example, there is an imbalance in the distribution of media coverage on relevant topics, and the coverage concentrates around World AIDS Day. The media agenda is also relatively negative in the overall agenda-setting process of the AIDS issue. Ultimately, media coverage generates a negative influence on the formation of public attitudes.

These problems prevent the media from effectively performing the functions in the process of solving the AIDS issue, which are precisely the social functions that the public media can and should assume. The problem may be due to socio-economic and cultural backgrounds with Chinese characteristics. In the specific socio-economic and cultural history, public media agenda setting is highly dependent on the policy agenda of the state sector.

Based on the above research, Dr. Chen concludes with some feasible recommendations to address the real problems in the media's construction of AIDS issues. The suggestions include improving the personal qualities of journalists, emphasising the demand for a public agenda and highlighting the primary role that the media should play in the construction of AIDS issues, in the resolution of AIDS issues and in the setting of media agenda.

Li (2009) argues that psychological changes occur in the early stages of public disclosure of HIV infection with the complete disintegration of social relationships. Influenced by stigmatisation systems of narrative discourse, the discrimination environment tends to be subjectively exaggerated. AIDS patients will experience a self-stigma, self-denial and self-isolation process. However, with the reconstruction of social relations, the publicity of AIDS knowledge and normalisation of the interaction and communication between infected and non-infected people, exaggerated environmental discrimination will be reversed and approach the real situation step by step.

In her thesis, Chunmei Li presents a comprehensive analysis of subjectively exaggerated environmental discrimination and explores the specific causes and possible ways of reversing or reverting to reality. Based on these analyses, Li points out that some necessary measures should be taken urgently to create a favourable living environment for PLWHA. These measures are suggested as follows. Firstly, to create a friendly living environment for PLWHA, the primary step is to change their subjectively constructed environment. Meanwhile, the public media should strive to publicise knowledge about HIV/AIDS and to produce fair reporting of HIV-related cases without intentional distortion. Secondly, to promote the return of PLWHA to rationality, it is necessary to change the hostile environment and to provide more psychological counselling for them. Thirdly, the communication between PLWHA and non-infected people should be promoted; that is, a normal and good way of interaction and communication should be established between the two groups, and isolation should be abandoned.

Chen (2007) exploits social constructionism as a theoretical paradigm, arguing that the HIV/AIDS issue not only exists as a social object or exists independently in a certain social context but in a more profound sense or in a sociological sense exists as a social process. Strictly speaking, the HIV/AIDS issue is a product of the interplay of individual and structural factors within a particular socio-economic and cultural context. This thesis examines the social construction of the AIDS problem in China at two levels: the construction of the AIDS problem by different social actors and the construction of the AIDS problem by socio-economic and cultural factors.

Zhang (2010) argues that the complicated connotations implied in the concept of AIDS are socially constructed, and in the course of a constructivist reading of the conceptual system of AIDS, he discusses the constructivist theory and details the constructivist view of illness, regarding illness as a functional definition, a value judgement and a social convention.

From a constructivist perspective, Dr. Zhang points out that stigmatisation is essentially a process of being labelled (e.g., based on moral judgments, HIV infection is caused by sexual promiscuity, which is typically a socially constructed process). Thus, what is "labelling"? It is an unequal treatment of PLWHA, an intentional alienation and rejection of groups or people with certain characteristics and attributes based on mainstream perceptions of society. In the theoretical context of social constructionism, "stigma" or "label", socially constructed, is the ultimate manifestation of social discrimination and social exclusion and is the result of the dominant group imposing norms and sanctions on the "offender", which is also socially constructed. It can be said that stigma and discrimination are mutually causal (this definition has limitations, as the causal relationship is unclear) or that it is difficult to determine which one is the cause or effect. It is in this sense that many social science researchers, including sociologists and psychologists, often use the terms "stigma" and "discrimination" as synonyms without giving specific interpretations and distinctions.

From a functionalist perspective, social discrimination, through disparagement, alienation and exclusion, imposes social sanctions of some degree on the social behaviours or social attributes negatively labelled. Stigma theory not only explains the inferiority of individuals and the distorted ideology that individuals harbor but also rationalises hostility based on class differences. In the sense of social construction theory, a type of social sanction or social discrimination reflects to some extent the intentional shaping of people's behaviour and thoughts by society in a particular economic and cultural-historical context, with the fundamental aim of stabilising established social norms and guaranteeing a particular social order. Social discrimination not only deprives discriminated people of the opportunity to participate in society but also inflicts greater economic loss on the group and, above all, exerts strong mental and psychological pressure. At the same time, such sanctions can lead them to associate their particular social behaviours and particular social attributes with their painful psychological and spiritual feelings. In short, discriminated people are forced to gradually correct their socially "deviant" behaviour or "shameful" attribute, a process that is quite tough.

2.1.2 Characteristics of Stigmatisation of People Living with HIV/AIDS

Hui Zhang (2004) analyses how China's dominant discourse of AIDS has developed and explores the possible effects of stigma on PLWHA and society. Her study discusses four main aspects: how PLWHA develop emotions or behaviours such as fear, concealment, resistance and retaliation; how they present AIDS as a serious threat that upsets their social life and reputation; how they try to hide their HIV-positive status as much as possible and resist being stigmatised; and how they are portrayed in the rumour as a group with a strong vengeful mood and social and psycho-psychological problems.

Dr. Xiaohu Zhang holds that social discrimination due to stigma is defined as the enforcement of social sanctions on discriminated people through social alienation and exclusion, and the aim of social discrimination is to ensure that established values, social norms and a particular social order are maintained and perpetuated. Dr. Zhang also distinguishes between two different types of social discrimination, namely, social discrimination for self-defence and social discrimination based on moral judgment, which reflect different standards of social judgement and have different social consequences.

The first type is called "social discrimination for self-defence", or fear-based social discrimination, which reflects the instinctive need for survival and the pursuit of health. The lack of knowledge about AIDS creates a psychological fear that leads to this type of discrimination. The second type is called "social discrimination based on moral judgment" or social discrimination due to "symbolic stigma". It reflects the social denouncement of "people at risk of AIDS" by the majority in a particular society or field in view of safeguarding traditional social values and social norms. This moral condemnation can also be described as social resistance and exclusion of non-mainstream values by mainstream values, which leads to the negative effect of the emotional experience of the excluded people and the emergence of a series of anti-social values and anti-social order behaviours. There are three main manifestations.

Firstly, there is an increase in psychological stress. The consequences of social discrimination not only exacerbate the psychological stress of PLWHA but also lead to the worsening of self-discrimination among them.

Secondly, they try to conceal HIV-positive status. As a result of the increasing psychological stress caused by social discrimination, PLWHA are aware of social disadvantages, the risk of disclosure, the loss of all social relationships, and difficult situations. Therefore, most of them choose to conceal their HIV-positive status to decrease the opportunity cost they should pay, especially when they realise the great probability of social discrimination.

The third one is about their resistance behaviour. When the mental, psychological and social pressure caused by social discrimination reaches a certain level, they are very likely to resort to extreme behaviours. The most extreme form of behaviour is social resistance; for example, some people may choose to commit suicide to end their mental and physical suffering. Other people may choose the method of "rights protection", which is becoming increasingly common as society progresses. There is another type of resistance that occurs in daily life, mainly because there is little social protection and care available to PLWHA at the level of social policy, the social discrimination and exclusion they suffer in certain social fields has not been improved, and their social situation remains unchanged. Like all social groups, PLWHA, the socially marginalised group, live in the real world, but the real world cannot be fully shaped or changed by social policies at the institutional level.

2.2 Research on the Needs of People Living with HIV/AIDS After Stigmatisation

2.2.1 Research on the "External" Needs of People Living with HIV/AIDS After Stigmatisation

PLWHA after stigmatisation have "external" needs and "internal" needs. Research on "external" needs, such as social support from government, community, family and friends, has been conducted using social surveys, social support theory, social exclusion theory or welfare pluralism theory. Studies on social support have mostly been conducted on PLWHA through blood transfusions, mostly from rural areas but also on people infected through sexual transmission, e.g., FSW (female sex workers) and MSM (men who have sex with men).

Research on this aspect focuses on the self-identity crisis that arises when PLWHA are stigmatised by society, media, institutions and organisations. In a situation of stigmatisation and social discrimination, PLWHA have a need for social support, recognition and help, either from the government, society, or the community or from relatives, friends and family members. From both social support and social adaptation, researchers have applied social surveys to study the status of social support in areas where HIV infection is severe. For example, Wu et al. (2006) conduct a cross-sectional study on the social support of PLWHA for blood-borne transmission in Anhui Province.

Li et al. (2007) argue that social support available to PLWHA includes various types of informal support within the family (moral and financial support and sharing of family responsibilities), support from friends, support at the community level, support from the public sphere at the government level, etc. The different levels of social support function differently for PLWHA. For example, family support can help to change their psychological states and improve their confidence in coping with the disease, while care and support from the public sector can help to reduce their mental stress and rekindle their hope in life. In short, there is no doubt that social support, no matter what level it comes from, helps them correct their self-perception.

Wu (2009) exploits a combination of quantitative and qualitative research methods to conduct a multi-level, multi-dimensional and multi-perspective comparative study on the social support and quality of life of PLWHA. The study of social support encompasses many dimensions, including personal support, support from the public sector, and support from various social organisations. The dimensions of social support for the AIDS community include both objective and subjective dimensions (needs and evaluations). Research perspectives on social support for PLWHA include sociocultural and social discrimination perspectives, as well as micro-social contexts, social capital theory and public policy perspectives.

2.2.2 *Research on the "Internal" Needs of People Living with HIV/AIDS After Stigmatisation*

The study of the "internal" needs of PLWHA after stigmatisation is mainly about their self-identity and emotion regulation. The HIV virus not only attacks the body of the infected person but also causes significant changes in their living environment and social support network. As a result, the social relationship and social support of PLWHA have suffered unprecedented damage, leading to a self-identity crisis and a crisis of belonging.

Meanwhile, in the context of social discrimination, social exclusion and social stigmatisation, PLWHA have no effective and legitimate ways to meet their needs for self-realisation and are at high risk of developing emotions such as shame, self-denial and even loneliness and anxiety. Due to the incurable nature of AIDS, they are at the risk of high mortality, which undoubtedly leads to their fear and despair.

The physical health and social relationships of PLWHA are of great significance in the construction of their own identity. Once individuals are infected with HIV, their physical conditions will change over time in stages. The public's understanding and awareness of HIV and infected people will likewise be further enhanced, and the public's attitude towards PLWHA will be transformed into the public sphere of society.

Chen (2013) argues that the identity status of PLWHA correlates with socio-demographic characteristics at the individual level and with socio-economic background. The identity of PLWHA is a socially constructed, dynamic process. Firstly, individuals construct social identity based on social categorisation, internalise it, and eventually complete self-identification. Secondly, individuals do not fully passively accept the identity constructed by society, and they do not accept it completely or develop a sense of belonging to a specific social group. In general, individuals construct their own identities through specific or a series of social interactions and through a strategic process, and their construction of the body in a specific socio-cultural context is one case.

Wu (2009) analyses the social support and survival quality of MSM, paid blood donors and FSW from the following perspectives: individual support, government support, organisational support and survival quality and social support of PLWHA, elucidating and comparing the structural characteristics of individual support, which mainly include the size, convergence and heterogeneity of the support network, the composition and strength of the relationship, and the social capital status of different social members in the network. In terms of the quality of survival and social support of PLWHA, the study analyses that the highest quality of survival is found among MSM, followed by paid blood donors, and the lowest is found among FWS.

Song (2012) argues that in the current social context of social discrimination, social exclusion and social stigma, the need for PLWHA for self-realisation cannot be attained through a legitimate approach; thus, they may experience shame, varying degrees of self-denial, and even loneliness and anxiety. The incurability of AIDS and the risk of high mortality rates can also lead to emotions of fear and despair at a psychological level.

2.3 Research on Assistance for People Living with HIV/AIDS After Stigmatisation

PLWHA need social assistance, which can help them adjust to negative emotions, eliminate anxiety, face reality and evoke hope in life.

2.3.1 Research on Assistance and Dilemmas of People Living with HIV/AIDS After Stigmatisation

Pengchao Li (2015) argues that the inadequacies of the practices of relevant departments and research institutions regarding the aid for PLWHA are mainly manifested in such aspects as the government's emphasis on prevention rather than aid, the lack of standardisation and sytematisation of institutional aid, academic research's emphasis on theory rather than practice, and inadequate coverage. The working model of Hong Kong's AIDS relief agencies works better in such aspects as the close cooperation of social workers, nurses, physiotherapists and fundraising teams and all-round services involving life, psychology, crisis intervention and personal development, which provide references for related work in the Chinese mainland.

Liu (2014) from Central China Normal University points out that social assistance for PLWHA through blood transfusions in central rural areas, out of touch with the actual situation, is not in line with their needs. The fracture in the implementation of social assistance policies has led to different forms of grassroots resistance by PLWHA in central rural areas. Fei Liu summarises the reasons for the fracture in the social assistance policy and the process and results of repairing it and then makes suggestions for improving the social assistance system and cultivating the subjectivity of PLWHA.

Xiang and Li (2010) discuss a new path to relieve AIDS patients from the social work perspective. At present, social assistance for PLWHA in China mainly focuses on the supply of relief resources and is not free from the influence of traditional relief methods. Overcoming these shortcomings requires the intervention of professional social work. They argue that social work functions significantly in social assistance for PLWHA and that social work is a new path to solve their psychological problems, restore their social relationships and enhance their social functioning. The theoretical basis for the intervention is discussed in terms of therapeutic, collectivist and reformist theories, followed by four models of social assistance: case work, group work, community work and social work administration.

Yu and Cheng (2006) analyse the economic, living, interpersonal and social difficulties faced by PLWHA through empirical surveys. In view of the predicament and demand of PLWHA, an improved social support system is rather important. The social support system should be built from three aspects: increasing publicity and creating a friendly living environment, establishing cooperation and support from various parties, and improving the service system. Li et al. (2007) analyse the status quo and needs from the perspective of improving the social support system for PLWHA and made suggestions that the social functions of NGOs (non-governmental organisations) should be given full play, the national "four frees and one care" policy should be improved, and social support networks for individuals should be improved so that PLWHA can receive the necessary social support.

2.3.2 Academic Research on the Relief for People Living with HIV/AIDS After Stigmatisation

There were studies on social support and social assistance for PLWHA after stigmatisation. Social support comes from the individual, the family, the community, the NGOs and the government. There were also studies on the human rights protection mechanism for PLWHA and introductions to the experience of providing relief for PLWHA in Hong Kong.

Xiang and Wu (2010) conduct a study on social support for PLWHA. In this study, they describe not only the structural characteristics of the social support network at the individual level but also the size, homogeneity and heterogeneity, composition of the network, strength of the relationship, and differences in the stock and quality of social capital among different social members of the social network. Based on these analyses, they further compare the differences in social relationship and social support networks among three different groups of PLWHA: MSM, paid blood donors and FSW, and conclude that the most social network capital possessed is found among MSM, followed by paid blood donors and FSW. In addition, the characteristics and problems faced by the three groups in terms of social support networks are discussed in the context of social capital and sociocultural discrimination.

They also claim that there are differences in the support and needs of different groups from government departments, as well as differences in their evaluation of government support. For example, for FSW, the needs and evaluations of policy support from the public sector were significantly lower than those of the other two groups. The differences may be related to both the level of resource scarcity and differences between groups in terms of social capital and awareness of rights; ultimately, the differences in satisfaction between groups may also be related to access to support and the level of satisfaction of needs.

At the same time, they analyse the problems in government support and the possible reasons. Firstly, social assistance policies vary across regions and populations; secondly, there are some problems in the distribution model of support resources for PLWHA in rural communities; thirdly, there are problems with the community-based social treatment and social assistance model; for example, there are differences in the restrictions on the household registration system between different communities and in health care resources between different primary health care institutions and designated health care institutions, which exerts a negative effect on their evaluation of government support.

In addition, organisational support for PLWHA is analysed mainly at three levels. Firstly, non-profit social organisations in HIV prevention and treatment are introduced, and the participation of three types of PLWHA in NGOs and in the subjective evaluation is compared. Secondly, through three NGOs as case studies, the participation of three different types of PLWHA in NGOs is analysed. Thirdly, the problems of the support from different NGOs and the reasons are discussed. The reasons discussed are as follows. Firstly, the competition for resources between different social organisations leads to differences in their fundraising capacity, and some organisations may even suffer from restrictions in this regard, which leads to a decrease in the trust of the organisations, and thus a decrease in the quality of the social organisations' support for PLWHA. Secondly, the social policy and legal system for NGOs in China need to be improved, and the policy and legal procedures have a deterrent effect on the support of NGOs. Thirdly, the social capital of different groups of PLWHA and the different levels of social policy control over them also have an impact on access to organisational support.

Finally, the study proposes solutions to the above problems, including accelerating the improvement and implementation of AIDS relief policies, strengthening the encouragement and support for the development of NGOs and further enhancing the organisational support for PLWHA. In terms of social awareness and social values, social discrimination and social rejection of PLWHA should be further reduced, and tolerance and humanistic care for the marginalised group should be enhanced.

2.3.3 Research on Social Problems Faced by People Living with HIV/AIDS After Stigmatisation at Home

The direct consequence of the stigmatisation of PLWHA is social exclusion. The manifestations of social stigmatisation of PLWHA are as follows.

Firstly, it manifests itself in the form of social discrimination against particular individuals or groups, for example, against people with physical disabilities or specific illnesses, or against a single gender, a certain class, a particular age or a particular ethnic group.

Secondly, there is social neglect and social deprivation of the fundamental rights of particular individuals and groups. Actually, this is a question about the social and cultural definition of humans. What does it truly mean to be human in a particular economic, social, cultural and historical context? In other words, what are the conditions that make "human"? How to define "human"? How to understand an individual, a group or subgroup? In the context of social construction theory, the formation of humans is a dynamic process of social construction that is not only embedded in the world of everyday life but also required to detach it from daily life.

Thirdly, stigma is not an abstract idea or abstract attitude in the minds of the public, and among the existing studies, some use quantitative research methods to measure stigma in the form of questionnaires and scales, while others use quantitative research methods complemented by qualitative ones, as stigma not only exists in the social sphere but also in family and private life. In short, stigma manifests itself in daily life and therefore requires observational and interpretive qualitative research using anthropological and sociological ethnographic methods.

Finally, another characteristic of stigmatisation is that stigma is embedded in everyday life. Individuals or groups suffer from it. How can research be conducted on their experience of stigma? Typically, two perspectives can be chosen: one is from the perspective of stigmatised people, i.e., PLWHA, and the second from the perspective of the perpetrators of stigma (e.g., from society, units, organisations and families). The studies, most from the perspective of the stigmatised, discuss their experiences of suffering to reveal the consequences of social stigma and its impact on the subjects involved. This second perspective is relatively scarce in existing research. The status quo of the research has led to a unidirectional and incomplete study on the experience of stigmatisation in domestic academia up to now, which obviously limits the in-depth exploration of the mechanisms that sustain the phenomenon of stigmatisation and the interpretive understanding of it in a sociological sense; this narrow research perspective has also led current academic research to understand or interpret the practice of stigma and institutionalised social discrimination and exclusion as simply the result or product of an inadequately informed and dysfunctional social mindset at the societal level. From the perspectives of governments, workplaces, social organisations and families, researchers have attempted to understand how PLWHA perceive and respond to non-infected people and the impact of HIV infection on their living environment, which is essential to a full understanding of the phenomenon of stigma and the mechanisms that sustain it and therefore cannot be ignored.

AIDS is undoubtedly a severely stigmatised disease, and there is widespread social discrimination of varied degrees against PLWHA in China. Social stigma and discrimination stem not only from fear of the disease itself but are also linked to a wider socio-economic and historical-cultural context. Although there are few studies at home that consider AIDS a socio-culturally constructed product in a sociological sense, this view is due to, or derives from, the production and reproduction of social culture. After the emergence of the "sexual revolution" in China, the "sexual transmission" of AIDS triggered massive "panic" in the social sphere. The social discrimination and social stigmatisation of PLWHA in the social sphere will not only have a negative impact on PLWHA but also pose a great threat and hindrance to the prevention and treatment of HIV at the social level, which will undoubtedly increase the potential threat of HIV to all areas of society. However, to date, there has been little systematic or in-depth research on the social stigma and discrimination of AIDS from the perspective of those who bear the stigma—PLWHA—as well as from their own experiences in the socio-economic and historical-cultural context of China. Therefore, this book focuses on an interpretive understanding, analysis and description of the complex implications of the oral histories of PLWHA of the social discrimination and social stigma and exclusion they have suffered.

2.3.4 Research on Social Problems Faced by People Living with HIV/AIDS After Stigmatisation Abroad

The research on the social problems faced by PLWHA after stigmatisation abroad has also undergone a historical process; after 1990, in the field of medical and anthropological studies, as the academic influence of critical perspectives grew, the concepts of social process, historical roots and social contexts in critical theory were gradually used in the study of stigmatisation and were constantly reinforced. Along with this, structural violence as a conceptual framework has been involved in the study of stigmatisation. During this period, a number of anthropologists from Haiti, Brazil and South Africa published representative works on the stigmatisation of AIDS.

Later, Kleinman (2007) proposes adding moral experience to stigma theory. Kleinman reveals that the common logic of historical acts against humanity, such as genocide, is that when in danger, humans tend to blame the danger on a particular "other", stigmatise it, and establish an alternative moral order. In such situations, humans often display extreme behavioural tendencies to protect their own safety. Social exclusion and violence, even destruction, against the stigmatised "other" are justified and legitimised. For Kleinman, stigmatisation implies not only the danger of moralisation but also justification and legitimisation, i.e., the process by which society as a whole justifies and legitimises the stigmatised "other" in an unequal, unfair and unjust way.

The anthropologist's study of stigmatisation offers two important and enlightening issues for subsequent researchers. Firstly, is it possible to understand stigma not from the perspective of particular individuals or groups of people? Is it possible to understand stigma from the universal phenomenon of human society? Secondly, how should subsequent researchers balance the current research favouring the object of stigmatisation? How can stigma be understood more deeply from a subject-construction perspective?

The vast majority of social psychologists have typically adopted social cognitive theory and focused on the causes of HIV stigma, with attribution theory being the most commonly used. According to Weiner (1988), the causative agent leads to a greater emotional response to PLWHA and further influences the attitudes and behaviour of the community towards them. Weiner argues that if the cause is uncontrollable, i.e., whether the person anticipates the consequences of their behaviour or not, then the public will be sympathetic towards the individuals as long as the causative behaviour is irresistible. This may, to a certain extent, lead to socially helpful behaviour by the community towards the individuals. However, if the causative agent of a particular disease is controllable, then the population in society will react more violently, and usually this emotional reaction tends to evolve into anger, and the general population will claim that the patient himself is responsible for his own actions, in which case the general population will adopt discriminatory attitudes and social behaviour towards the patient.

Mak et al. (2006) argue that attribution theory could be allowed for the psychological clarification of the mechanisms that shape the phenomenon of stigma, which has been recognised by most researchers and applied to the study of stigmatisation against various illnesses.

Parker and Aggleton (2003) reconstruct the conceptual framework of stigma from the sociocultural perspective, arguing that the concept of stigma is ambiguous and deviates from the classic definition of stigma proposed by Goffman. According to Goffman (1963), stigma is ultimately an attribute that lowers an individual's social status. The process of stigmatising others is the construction of hierarchies and notions of social order within society as a whole to elevate the social status of the dominant group, and the further use of institutionalisation to legitimise and legalise these hierarchies and orders. From a critical perspective, attribution theory places too much emphasis on the study of the individual, on individual perceptions and on the impact of individual perceptions on social interactions. However, attribution theory overlooks the fact that social stigma and discrimination are sociocultural phenomena linked to humanity as a whole and cannot simply be attributed to individuals. Parker (2003), citing the French philosopher Foucault and the sociologist Bourdieu on social power and social culture, explains that stigma lies at the crossroads of social culture, power and different groups and that stigma and discrimination not only manifest themselves in differences but also become more explicitly associated with elements of inequality at the level of social structure. Stigmatising others is thus the manifestation of a complex struggle for power in social life, with some people gaining social power and access to high-quality social resources through socially constructed institutions or hegemony. Meanwhile, the stigmatisation of others continues, with the group achieving dominance through social structural inequalities and finding ways to make the dominance more legitimate.

The socio-cultural theory is another theory that is more widely used. Yang et al. (2007) propose a conceptual model of stigma based on the theory, arguing that the core feature of stigma is that people may feel that certain spiritual aspects they cherish (such as reputation, dignity, etc.) are at risk of imminent loss. In a given social context, the public stigmatises others in response to perceived danger or to real danger and fear of the unknown, not only as a mechanism of self-protection and psychological defence for the stigmatised but also on the level of moral evaluation.

However, for stigmatised individuals, stigma undoubtedly causes suffering, which is gradually compounded. That is, the stigmatised individual is confronted not only with his or her own undisclosed status but also with confusion, such as diminished social status and damaged social reputation. The cross-cultural similarity of stigmatisation, according to Major and O'Brien (2005), can be defined as a cognitive adaptation at the societal level that has developed in the course of social evolution, through social discrimination and exclusion, to isolate those who have or may have certain undesirable traits or who do not conform to established social norms to avoid the potential risks of living in groups.

Yang et al. (2007) apply the conceptual model of stigma to the area of "face" in the Chinese context, synthesising recent research on stigma in China in relation to PLWHA and schizophrenia to propose three different levels of social stigma and use these models to explain the processes and mechanisms by which the social characteristics of stigma are produced. These models are used to explain the processes and mechanisms by which social features of stigma are created. At the top level are the social factors that influence stigma, including public perceptions and social institutions. The former includes stereotypes of the general public about AIDS, reflecting the hierarchy of society. The latter represents the economic, political, historical and cultural aspects of society; these two aspects are macro factors that objectively determine AIDS stigma, which is similar to the explanations in social and cultural theory. The second layer of the model concerns the morality of stigma. The moral evaluation of AIDS has changed considerably with the development of society and technological advances, especially the increasing awareness of rights. However, being infected with HIV is still "losing face" for individuals, and the status of being infected deprives them of social resources. The third level contains three separate and interrelated elements that together act as a correlative mechanism for the impact of stigma on individuals. At the subjective level, changes in morality have a dynamic effect on changes in mood. Loss of reputation in the moral system usually leads to emotional depression, but moral changes in stigma can lead to profound changes in the physiological level of the individual.

At the collective level, stigmatisation from society is a social phenomenon that occurs between family members or within social networks. We know that "losing face" is a collective feeling because of the shame felt by the whole family or the whole social network when the identity of the infected person is made public (not even to mention to others any information about the infected person). This stigma from the collective level of society is the result and presentation of the whole social construction and interaction. For example, the stigmatisation of health care and family members is prevalent in social reality during the stigmatisation of AIDS. Furthermore, relational capital or, to use a sociological concept, the lack of social capital is also caused by the termination or difficulty of interpersonal relationships. In the specific case of PLWHA, this lack of interpersonal or social capital may manifest itself in the institutionalised discrimination and exclusion of PLWHA from the social system in the social processes of living, working and learning, such as job hunting, accommodation renting, and re-education receiving.

2.4 Theoretical Foundations

2.4.1 Social Exclusion Theory

2.4.1.1 Literature Review on Social Exclusion Abroad

(1) The Emergence and Development of Social Exclusion

In the course of human history, social exclusion emerges very early. There was the system of "ostracism" in the ancient Greek city-state period, the system of "capitis deminutio" in the ancient Roman Empire, and the long-standing "caste system" in Indian society. However, it is only in recent times that "social exclusion" has been studied and analysed in depth. Social exclusion is derived from the study of social poverty, which was prominent in the process of social transformation in Europe.

In 1974, René Lenoir, then Secretary of State for Social Action in a French Gaullist government, first used the term in *Les Exclus: Un Francais sur Dix*. He spoke of the following as constituting the "excluded"—a tenth—of the French population: mentally and physically handicapped, suicidal people, aged invalids, abused children, substance abusers, delinquents, single parents, multi-problem households, marginal, asocial persons, and other social "misfits". The notion has already made substantial inroads into the discussions and writings on poverty and deprivation.

In the 1980s, the concept of "social exclusion" was used by the Commission of the European Communities to analyse poverty, as social exclusion encompasses the basic human rights of citizens. In the 1990s, with the accelerated pace of economic globalisation in Western countries, particularly in Europe, business competition became more intense, and industrial consolidation, restructuring and mergers took place at a feverish pace. While these initiatives promoted economic development, they also led to massive structural unemployment, the creation of new classes of poor people and the emergence of various socially marginalised groups (beggars, thieves, etc.) as a result of poverty. In this context, the concept of "social exclusion" became widespread in academia, and a systematic theory of social exclusion was developed.

(2) Social Exclusion, Social Discrimination and Social Problems Induced

On the basis of Lenoir's research, the specific connotations and extensions of social exclusion theory from different perspectives have been studied in depth. For example, British sociologist Anthony Giddens (1998) points out that an individual may encounter social exclusion of different levels, depending on their social status and class.

American sociologist Popenoe (1999) argues from the perspective of ethnic groups that the dominant group or large ethnic group that holds the monopoly of resources in society discriminates against other groups or ethnic minorities.

Social discrimination is a term closely related to social exclusion. For example, age discrimination. It is a general term that refers to negative stereotypes and derogatory evaluations of a certain age group, where the discriminated individual is more likely to be deprived of equal access to opportunities, resources and treatment of all kinds. Age discrimination is more common in older people, and it is a means of denying or violating the human rights of older people. The prevailing negative stereotypes and devaluation of older people lead to social indifference, marginalisation and isolation, making it more difficult for them to enjoy their rights equally.

Ageism is a stereotype or inherent prejudice against older people who exaggerates their certain negative characteristics. According to Palmore (1999), ageism is based on plausible judgements but inaccurate facts. Ageism, which appears in all walks of life, mostly occurs in the field of labour employment, where older workers may be excluded due to their age. Seniors have no equal access to suitable jobs because of their age and not their ability. The elimination of age discrimination is significant in addressing social equity between different age groups. With the rapid development of modernisation and the market economy, ageism has given rise to a great deal of social injustice, such as job opportunities, job promotion and the distribution of benefits, evaluated by the mere rigid setting of age criteria rather than qualifications, thus resulting in a huge waste of human resources and seriously dampening human motivation.

A glance at the legal policies of some developed countries will reveal that an increasing number of studies of social equality are being adopted by governments and reflected in their laws and institutions. For example, research on this area in the United States has contributed to the legislation of *The Age Discrimination in Employment Act*. There are a number of social consequences associated with social discrimination. In the case of ageism, for example, some studies have pointed out that at the extreme end of the spectrum, ageism can lead to elder abuse (including cases materially unsupported and poorly cared for). As the economy develops, traditional filial culture is being ignored, and society is in moral decline. Most of the elderly are given material support but no companionship or care, and they even suffer physical and mental abuse, which directly affects their physical and mental health. The problems of elder abuse cannot be solved by the law alone and need to be studied and addressed in the context of comprehensive social governance.

There are various definitions of "elder abuse". The widely accepted one provided by the United Nations holds that elder abuse is a single or repeated act, occurring within any relationship where there is an expectation of trust, which causes harm or distress to an older person without taking appropriate actions. With the growing interest in human rights issues around the world, awareness of the rights of older people has also grown, especially since the United Nations General Assembly in 1982 in Madrid, and ageing issues have been gradually recognised as human rights. The focuses are as follows: the political implications of elder abuse and discrimination; the means and acts of depriving older people of their economic and social rights; and measures and recommendations to stop abuse and violence.

Elder abuse can occur in the home, the community, institutions, and the workplace, and the identification of elder abuse is becoming clearer and more specific as research progresses, but regardless of the type of abuse, it violates the internationally agreed rights of older people.

Relative or absolute economic poverty, disadvantage in political power and progressive marginalisation in social participation can all lead to elder abuse. It is therefore argued that the global issue of elder abuse can only be successfully addressed when people's basic needs and rights are met throughout all stages of the life cycle. However, the abuse of older people is difficult to address properly in reality, and this difficulty arises first and foremost from the difficulty of recognising abuse. The elimination of elder abuse depends on political commitment and legal safeguards.

How can social discrimination exist in society and the consequences induced, and how can social discrimination and the negative consequences be eliminated in light of social institutions? The following is research into the elimination of age discrimination and elder abuse.

The Universal Declaration of Human Rights (UDHR), adopted by the United Nations General Assembly in 1948, enshrines the rights and freedoms of all human beings. Everyone is entitled to all the rights in the political, social, economic and cultural spheres, manifesting the spirit of freedom, equality and human rights, which shows that all are equal. To a large extent, the UDHR forms the basis of international legislation on rights. The development of population ageing has reinforced the international community's awareness of and attention to the rights of older people. By the middle of the twentieth century, population ageing had already attracted a great deal of attention from many countries, and it is at the urging of these countries that the first World Assembly on Ageing was held in Vienna in 1982, which culminates in the adoption of the *Vienna International Plan of Action on Ageing* that outlines the rights of older people. This conference reaffirms that the fundamental rights in UDHR should be fully applicable to older age groups.

However, following the adoption of the *Vienna International Plan of Action on Ageing*, many countries soon found that the situation of older people varied greatly not only from country to country but also within countries and among individuals, requiring a diversity of policies. To encourage governments to involve some of the principles of older people in their national programmes, the United Nations General Assembly, convened in December 1991, gave full recognition to the contribution of older people to society, affirmed the fundamental human rights, dignity and worth of the human person in the *Charter of the United Nations*, and further emphasised the importance of *UDHR*, *International Covenant on Economic, Social and Cultural Rights* and *International Covenant on Civil and Political Rights*, as well as other declarations. *The United Nations Principles for Older Persons*, adopted in 1991, identifies independence, participation, care, self-fulfillment and dignity as fundamental principles for older persons.

The United Nations Principles for Older Persons ensures the fundamental rights and goals to be achieved by older people. Even though countries differ in their level of socio-economic development and their cultural and historical backgrounds, their policies, laws and measures relating to older persons should guarantee the achievement of these fundamental principles. Independence in *the United Nations Principles for Older Persons* refers not only to financial and material security and safety in the living environment but also to real independence and freedom through education and work to improve one's abilities. The principle of participation, for older persons, means participating actively in the formulation and implementation of policies that directly affect their well-being and share their knowledge and skills with younger generations and form movements or associations of older persons. For the principle of care, older persons should have access to health care to help them maintain or regain the optimum level of physical, mental and emotional well-being and to prevent or delay the onset of illness. Older persons should have access to social and legal services to enhance their autonomy, protection and care. Older persons should be able to enjoy human rights and fundamental freedoms when residing in any shelter, care or treatment facility, including full respect for their dignity, beliefs, needs and privacy and for the right to make decisions about their care and the quality of their lives. For the principle of self-fulfillment, older persons should be able to pursue opportunities for the full development of their potential and have access to the educational, cultural, spiritual and recreational resources of society. In terms of the principle of dignity, older persons should be able to live in dignity and security, be free of exploitation and physical or mental abuse, be treated fairly regardless of age, gender, racial or ethnic background, disability or other status, and be valued independently of their economic contribution. It can be said that the introduction of the UN Principles is a manifestation of consensus on the human rights of older people and an enhancement of the international community's understanding of the rights of older people, giving different countries a clearer direction and goal in dealing with population ageing and addressing the problems of older people.

To raise awareness, promote research and strengthen policy implementation worldwide, the United Nations General Assembly observed 1999 as the International Year of Older Persons (IYOP). The theme of IYOP is towards a society for all ages, implying that equality and sharing should be embodied in groups of all ages and that they should not be excluded because of ageing. It can be said that the above-mentioned policy document is an important guide for the introduction of policy measures and programmes of action to limit social discrimination and social exclusion and their related social consequences, both at the international level and at the level of specific countries and regions worldwide.

2.4.1.2 Research on Social Exclusion at Home

There are various definitions of social exclusion in China. The first view emphasises the process of exclusion and regards social exclusion as a process whereby individuals, groups and organisations are excluded from economic, political, family and social relationships and social systems due to the interests of agents such as the state, corporations and interest groups.

The second view holds that social exclusion is the result of institutions and policies. For example, Tang (2002) claims that social exclusion is based on strong institutional planning and policy formulation and that the purpose of conducting social policy research is to point out the flaws in the current situation so that by improving or even changing these unreasonable parts, they can be made fair and reasonable and benefit all members of society.

The third view believes that the disadvantageous position of citizens leads to social exclusion. This disadvantageous position, due to its own factors or policy reasons or both, makes the disadvantaged group lack the opportunity to participate fairly in society and eventually be detached from social mainstream. For example, Yang (2002) argues that the exclusion caused by disadvantageous status is a persistent and dynamic process, resulting in bond breaking in civil society. Shi Tong, on the other hand, argues that certain individuals, families or groups are marginalised or isolated due to a lack of opportunities to participate in social activities.

2.4.2 Stigma Theory

Stigma is widespread in the society. The main subjects of stigma research are people with Parkinson's syndrome, blind people, cancer patients, children, drug addicts, heart patients, paraplegics, obese people, PLWHA and homosexuals. Stigma is a common phenomenon in social psychology, and many psychologists have defined stigma from different perspectives.

Stigma is typically explained as "a mark of shame, a sense of shame". Stigma, from Latin, first referred to the "mark made on skin by burning with a hot iron" to indicate a low social status. Later, the term came to be used as a metaphor for physical defects or a mark of disgrace. This significance of "stigma" is undoubtedly negative, representing a range of attributes that should be rejected by society, such as "shame" and "humiliation". In a given social context, a person with such attributes is often supposed to be "reduced to a flawed, despised person".

In 1963, Goffman introduced "stigma" into the field of psychology. For Goffman, a stigma is an attribute, behaviour, or reputation that is socially discrediting in a particular way: it causes an individual to be mentally classified by others in an undesirable, rejected stereotype rather than in an accepted, normal stereotype. In Goffman's view, the word "stigma" represents a deeply humiliating characteristic or attribute, not only as a derogatory and insulting symbol and label for these individuals and marginalised groups in society but also as a representation of a defect such as a physical disability or even a stain on an individual's character qualities or as an unpopular marginalised class or membership of a group that is different from the dominant group in a society. Typically, the labelled individual will have attributes, qualities or behavioural characteristics that are not accepted by social mainstream, and the group will often experience subjective feelings of shame, stigma or a sense of guilt about the social attributes or social behaviour they possess because of these labels. The rest will experience injustice towards the group as a result, and the accumulation of such injustices can lead to social exclusion and social discrimination.

By definition, stigmatised people are assumed to be abnormal. Based on this assumption, they are discriminated in a number of ways that, even if not intentionally, can lead to loss of opportunities for survival and development to some extent.

Stigma often manifests itself as social discrimination. The word "discrimination" is interpreted as suffering "unfair treatment", which is a form of alienation, restriction, exclusion or even, in a general sense, social abandonment of certain people and groups that are perceived as having negative attributes and are socially marginal. The word "qishi" in Chinese can be used not only as an English verb "discriminate" but also as the noun "discrimination". As an act of discrimination, it typically refers to discrimination against people who, in general, tend to have a negative label or stigma or who are stigmatised by social mainstream. The concept of discrimination connotes a variety of negative attitudes and behavioural orientations towards people labelled as stigmatised, such as attitudes and behaviours that are demeaning, alienating or, to some extent, hostile towards the group. Discrimination can be described as the result of "stigmatisation".

Western sociologists have interpreted the theory of stigma from two perspectives, collectivism and individualism, and the diversity of research perspectives has undoubtedly deepened the understanding of stigma as a social phenomenon.

On the one hand, among the studies based on the collectivist perspective, Elias (1994) is the first sociologist to put forward the concept of stigmatisation. In his study of Huguenots, he found a social process and phenomenon; that is, the mainstream group imposes the inferiority of human nature on the marginalised group and reinforces the process through specific social institutions. Simply speaking, stigmatisation essentially reflects social power relations regarding the one-way "naming", which exists between two social groups, not only in terms of their social interaction but also in terms of the difference in social impressions imposed on the marginalised group and the special relationship between the two groups. It is important to note that the process of social stigmatisation is an evolving process of interaction between the two groups and a practical process of solidifying social phenomena and social facts. It should be noted in particular that Goffman, in his classic study, explains stigmatisation as an undesirable attribute possessed by an individual, which is denied by members of the dominant group. In extreme cases, these individuals are considered by the dominant group to be bad, dangerous or weak. The stigmatised persons are considered to be relegated to those with tainted and discredited personalities, which gives the marginal group a generally stigmatising trait. For this reason, Goffman divides stigmatised people into three categories: "First, there are abominations of the body—the various physical deformities. Next, there are blemishes of individual characters perceived as weakly ill, domineering or unnatural passions, treacherous and rigid beliefs, and dishonesty, which are inferred from a known record of, for example, mental disorder, imprisonment, addiction, alcoholism, homosexuality, unemployment, suicidal attempts, and radical political behaviour. Finally, there are the tribal stigma of race, nation, and religion, these being stigma that can be transmitted through lineages and equally contaminate all members of a family" (1963: 4).

Goffman places stigmatisation at the core of social construction and abstracts stigma itself as a particular relationship between the characteristics of mainstream society and rigid dogma, a relationship rooted in a linguistic relationship in which stigma embodies a certain heterogeneity between real social identities in a social situation. In contrast to Goffman, Jones et al. (1984) define the stigmatised person as a bearer of a mark that defines him or her as deviant, flawed, limited, spoiled or generally undesirable; they describe stigmatisation as a process of social relations and social interaction, i.e., it can be the social environment that is used to define an individual's deviant or transgressive behaviour. It is further argued that the essence of stigma is a psychosocial mechanism and a psychosocial process. In their conceptualisation, Link and Phelan (2001) suggest that stigma exists when the following interrelated components converge: labelling, stereotyping, separation, status loss, and discrimination co-occur in a power situation. It is important to note that the first four are social processes that occur within the socio-historical and cultural context in which the individual or group is embedded. Social discrimination, on the other hand, includes structural social discrimination, which refers to the institutional arrangements from society as a whole that disadvantage stigmatised groups. In sum, the concepts of stigma used by the above scholars in their respective studies are unique in pointing out that the process of stigmatisation relies on or draws on social, economic and even socio-political forces and that the presence of these forces constitutes a subversive and even discriminatory and serious consequence for the first four components of stigmatisation.

On the other hand, in studies using an individualist perspective, there is no doubt that the stigmatised individual is also a focus of considerable importance. Social psychologists often choose to regard stigma as an attribute of an individual. However, Crocker et al. (1998) argue that stigmatisation occurs when the individual possesses attributes or when the individual is characterised by a socially devalued status in a particular social context. Through this process, stigmatised identity is naturally socially constructed and developed. Like the sociologist Goffman, Crocker argues that stigma is discrediting in a sociological sense. However, in the specific course of its study, it does not focus exclusively on a particular individual or individuals who are stigmatised but insists that the reason why stigmatisation occurs and suffers derogation is the consequence in a particular social context.

2.4.3 Actor Theory

Strictly speaking, actor theory belongs to the realm of philosophical topics, which deals with the whole range of human consciousness and behaviour. It can be traced back to the Aristotelian period, with Nicomachean ethics as its historical starting point. After this, theories of action were gradually incorporated into the social sciences. With the advent and development of psychology and neuroscience, many of the theories of action have been confirmed by experiments.

The term "actor" is traditionally regarded by society as belonging exclusively to human beings and as a concrete expression of human initiative. Actor theory, however, poses a subversive challenge to this understanding. French sociologists first proposed actor-network theory, in which the subjects of actors include not only human beings but also non-human beings or forces, in addition to a mixture of different types of material and immaterial things (Callon, 1986; Latour, 1987). After this, the

American philosopher Harman (2013) developed an in-depth study of actor-network theory, and his specific research route is to develop the concept of "object-oriented philosophy". What is the concept of "object-oriented philosophy"? This means that any person or any object can be the subject or the protagonist, thus providing a philosophical interpretation for the legitimacy and justification of the Actant. Following the research and critical development of the above-mentioned scholars, actor theory has been widely applied in many fields of social science research in the following decades. To a large extent, it can be argued that actor theory can help research by bringing researchers back into the larger picture of "everything is an actor", using the functional word "action" that is distinctly dynamic, rather than just "being" that is distinctly static. From this perspective, it is clear that all things, whether they are people or things, can be actors. On this basis, the measure of the actor lies in the process of action and the consequences of the act itself.

The famous French sociologist Latour (1987) extends the concept of the actor from the social sciences to the natural sciences. For Latour, social networks include both human actors and non-human actors and the will of these non-human actors, which is, in general, expressed through agents. In this process, an actor network is the process by which heterogeneous actors build and develop networks through which they solve particular social problems; it is not only a dynamic process but can also be described as a static social fact. Within the framework of actor network theory, science, as an important dimension, also evolves into science in social action, in which the science of social action reshapes the social structure and social order. In this sense, we can say that Latour organically combined the perspectives of relational and process thinking. His success in introducing both into the process of analysing scientific facts not only greatly expands the horizons of later participants in scientific research but also suggests a new direction for future research in the sociology of science and technology.

Studies on actor theory mostly focus on the causes and processes of human behaviour in relation to cause and effect, as well as the mechanisms by which the stigmatisation of PLWHA is affected, the ways in which social structures inherently shape the discrimination and stigma of PLWHA, the hitherto incurable nature of HIV and its inextricable link to sex from its discovery. The theory demonstrates how AIDS influences governmental, social and civil attitudes towards AIDS and how it amplifies the effect of stigmatisation. In terms of social actors, the study selected not only PLWHA but also the mass media and the government as the three representative groups as objects of the study. The study also specifically examines the role of PLWHA in the construction of their own identity and in the construction of the media discourse on AIDS, as well as the government's balance between public interest and personal interest. Finally, the study points out that in the absence of PLWHA, powerful discourses from the media and the government have a profound impact on the formation of public attitudes towards HIV.

2.4.4 *Theory of Welfare Pluralism*

2.4.4.1 The Definition of Welfare Pluralism

Welfare pluralism typically refers to the mixed economy of social welfare—the myriad sectors through which consumers encounter services. In other words, welfare pluralism advocates a plurality of providers of social welfare. This plurality of sources not only emphasises that welfare should not be entirely dependent on the market or on the public sector of the state but that welfare should also be a product of society as a whole. More specifically, the provision of welfare requires not only the commitment of the state but also the active participation of civil society.

Specifically, there are four main providers: the state, the private sector, the voluntary sector and informal provision. In addition, there are more providers. The higher the level of overall social welfare is, the more it demands providers of welfare provision.

As early as 1978, the term "welfare pluralism" appeared in the British report "The Future of Voluntary Organisations", which proposed that voluntary organisations should also be included as welfare providers and that welfare pluralism should be applied to social policy in Britain, giving full play to the role of ideas and theories in guiding social practice.

Firstly, Rose (1986) provides a detailed definition of welfare pluralism in "Common Goals but Different Roles: The State's Contribution to the Welfare Mix". Ross first clarifies the basic concept of the welfare state. Then, he argues that the welfare state, although well known, is an ambiguous concept, especially as it is very easily misconceived and belongs exclusively to the participation of the public sector. There is no doubt that the state should indeed play an important role in the major matter of providing social welfare, but it should also never have a complete monopoly on social welfare.

Secondly, Ross argues that total welfare in society is the sum of the household (family), market and state. It would be biased to exclude the source of the market and the family, the two main welfare providers outside the public sector of the state, and to leave it to the state to assume full responsibility for welfare provision in a modern, fast-moving society. The sum of the household (family), market and state, i.e., total social welfare, can be expressed in the formula TWS = HXMXS. In this equation, TWS refers to total social welfare, H household provider, M market provider and S state provider. In modern society, the state is, as a rule, the primary provider of welfare, but that does not mean that it is the only provider. Outside the state, the market is undoubtedly one of the sources of social welfare in general because in modern society, for each of us, both individuals and families, we have to buy from the market all kinds of material and spiritual goods related to our daily life. Additionally, from the point of view of historical development and social evolution, the family has always been one of the basic providers of social welfare, its functions were also diverse in the pre-industrial era, and this diversity was able to meet the diverse needs of the different members of the family.

Thirdly, the market, the state and the household are all deficient to some extent if they act alone as welfare providers. The three sectors should work together to complement each other and avoid their weaknesses, which is in line with the inherent requirements of welfare pluralism. For example, the state provision is, to some extent, intended to avoid "market failures"; the state's monopoly on the provision of social welfare resources as a whole may lead to "government failures" and attract criticism from the social sphere. At the same time, the state provision and the household provision, to a certain extent, aim to avoid "family failures", while the household provision and the voluntary provision, such as voluntary organisations, are, to a certain extent, intended to compensate for deficiency of provision from the market and the state.

Finally, a welfare society with multiple providers is one in which the growth of social welfare provided by the state, to a certain extent or within a certain range, does not completely exclude the growth of social welfare provided by households and the market. When the social benefits provided by these three actors are all increasing at the same time, we can say that society with multiple providers is created. In this pluralist society, social groups are able to recognise not only the importance of the state as a fiscal benefit but also the self-evident importance of the contribution of the market and the family to social welfare. In short, in the theoretical perspective of welfare pluralism, the state, the market and the family are not so much in competition with each other as they are in complementarity with each other, and the growth of one does not entirely replace the contribution of the others to overall social welfare.

2.4.4.2 Core Elements of Welfare Pluralism

In the research on social policy, welfare pluralism emphasises that social welfare and services should be provided by multiple sectors: state provision and private provision. This means that state provision, which has traditionally been dominant in society, should be reduced in contemporary society and that the provision of welfare should change as soon as possible from a situation dominated by a monopolistic organisation or public sector to a more diversified and competitive one. To be more specific, there are two core elements of welfare pluralism: pluralism and decentralisation.

Firstly, as stated above, pluralism means that there should be multiple sources of social welfare in general, including not only the state but also market actors such as enterprises, families, voluntary organisations, communities and other social actors, which are also important sources of social welfare. To effectively address the social crisis that exists in the welfare state, attention should be given to the important role that social sectors other than the government can play and should play in the process of social welfare provision. It is in this sense that welfare pluralism argues for a shift from the practice of having the government sector take over the provision of social welfare to the introduction of provision from the market, the family and other social organisations. Social welfare can be provided not only by government departments, voluntary organisations, the business sector and other informal sectors but also by these sectors according to their own characteristics and strengths, providing various types of diversified social welfare to the public. As we know, in the current social practice, in the transformation of many welfare states into a pluralist welfare portfolio, the core of the transformation is "privatisation" and "non-government", that is to say, the importance of the transformation is to reduce the role of the government.

Secondly, in terms of decentralisation, the provision of social welfare and services should, as soon as possible, change from the previous situation where the central or local government public sector was the sole provider or provider of all services to a situation where smaller regional or social organisations are responsible for as much as possible. The essence of decentralisation, as emphasised by social welfare theory, lies in the emphasis on the localisation of social welfare and services, on the community dimension of social welfare and services, on the active participation and actual choice of consumers in the process of social welfare and service provision, and therefore, in this sense, decentralisation also has a strong anti-stratification as well as a strong anti-specialisation dimension.

The destigmatisation of PLWHA should be analysed from the perspective of welfare pluralism, seeking the support and cooperation of the government, the community, civil society organisations and PLWHA themselves, bringing into play the joint role of multiple subjects, building bridges of communication between them, eliminating the effects of stigmatisation and its negative consequences, creating a good living environment for PLWHA.

References

Callon M (1986) The sociology of an actor-network: the case of the electric Vehicle. In: Callon M, Law J, Rip A (eds) Mapping the dynamics of science and technology: sociology of science in the real world. Macmillan

Chen J (2013) The research on self-identity of AIDS patients: a case study of AIDS patients in HL village the Northwest of Hubei [Master's thesis, Wuhan University]. CNKI. https://kns.cnki.net/KCMS/detail/detail.aspx?dbname=CMFD201401&filename=1013276141.nh

Chen ML (2012) An empirical study of the media construction about the issue of AIDS—an agenda-setting perspective [PhD thesis, Wuhan University]. CNKI. https://kns.cnki.net/KCMS/detail/detail.aspx?dbname=CDFD1214&filename=1013117239.nh

Chen Y (2007) A study of the social construction process of AIDS in China [Master's thesis, Kunming University of Technology]. CNKI. https://kns.cnki.net/KCMS/detail/detail.aspx?dbname=CMFD2008&filename=2008111458.nh

Crocker J, Major B, Steele C (1998) Social stigma. In: Fiske S, Gilbert D, Lindzey G (eds) Handbook of social psychology. McGraw-Hill

Elias N, Scotson JL (1994) The established and the outsiders, 2nd ed. SAGE

Giddens A (1998) The third way and its critics. Polity

Goffman E (1963) Stigma; notes on the management of spoiled identity. Prentice-Hall

Harman G (2013) An outline of object-oriented philosophy. Sci Progress Rev J Current Sci Adv 96(2):187–199

Jones EE, Farina A, Hastorf AH, Markus H, Miller DT, Scott RA (1984) Social stigma: the psychology of marked relationships. Freeman

Latour B (1987) Science in action: how to follow scientists and engineers through society. Harvard University Press

Lenoir R (1974) Les exclus: un Francais sur dix. Le Seuil

Li C (2009) The study of AIDS patients' subjective construction of discrimination environment [Master's thesis, Central China Normal University]. CNKI. https://kns.cnki.net/KCMS/detail/detail.aspx?dbname=CMFD2009&filename=2009159691.nh
Li P (2015) The model and implication of Hong Kong AIDS patients relief: field study of a Hong Kong institution. Social Work Manage 1:33–39
Li X, Ma Y, Li S, Hu C (2007) Social support systems for PLWHA. Med Philos (A) 06:28–29
Link BG, Phelan JC (2001) Conceptualizing stigma. Ann Rev Sociol 27:363–385
Liu F (2014) Fracture and repair: AIDS patients and social assistance policy—the case: S village in H Province [PhD thesis, Central China Normal University]. CNKI. https://kns.cnki.net/KCMS/detail/detail.aspx?dbname=CMFD201402&filename=1014239688.nh
Mak WWS, Mo PKH, Cheung RYM, Woo J, Cheung FM, Lee D (2006) Comparative stigma of HIV/AIDS, SARs, and tuberculosis in Hong Kong. Soc Sci Med 63:1912–1922
Major B, O'Brien LT (2005) The social psychology of stigma. Annu Rev Psychol 56:393–422
Palmore E (1999) Ageism: negative and positive, 2nd ed. Springer
Parker R, Aggleton P (2003) HIV and AIDS-related stigma and discrimination: a conceptual framework and implications for action. Soc Sci Med 57:13–24
Popenoe D (1986) Sociology, 11th ed. Prentice-Hall
Rose R (1986) Common goals but different roles: the state's contribution to the welfare mix. In: Rose R, Shiratori R (eds) The welfare state east and west. Oxford University Press
Shi T (2002) The theoretical significance of the study of gender exclusion. Collect Women's Stud 4:17–25
Song X (2012) A study on emotion regulation of AIDS patients: a case study of Wuhan city [PhD thesis, Wuhan University]. CNKI. https://kns.cnki.net/KCMS/detail/detail.aspx?dbname=CMFD2012&filename=1012386237.nh
Tang J (2002) The primary goal of social policy: eliminating poverty and social rejection. Jiangsu Social Sci 3:41–47
Weiner B, Perry RP, Magnusson J (1988) An attributional analysis of reactions to stigmas. J Pers Soc Psychol 55:738–748
Wu D (2009) Social support and quality of life of PLWHA: a comparative study on paid blood donors, MSM and FSW [PhD thesis, Wuhan University]. CNKI. https://kns.cnki.net/KCMS/detail/detail.aspx?dbname=CDFD1214&filename=1011071138.nh
Wu H, Sun Y, Wu R et al (2006) The cross-sectional study on the social support of PLWHA for blood-borne transmission in Jingjiu township of Fuyang city of Anhui Province. Modern Prev Med 33:2227–2230
Xiang D, Li G (2010) Social work: a new path to relieve AIDS patients. Henan Social Sci 18(1):122–125
Xiang D, Wu D (2010) A comparative study between AIDS patients' social support and life quality: empirical survey of paid blood group, MSM group and FSWs. Social Sci Front 4:194–200
Yang LH, Kleinman A, Link BG, Phelan JC, Lee S, Good B (2007) Culture and stigma: adding moral experience to stigma theory. Soc Sci Med 64(7):1524–1535
Yang T (2002) Evolution of the research paradigm of social policy and its enlightenment to us. Social Sci China Press 4:127–139
Yu Y, Cheng L (2006) Difficulty need and social support of the AID/HIV patients. J Publ Health Prev Med 17(5):20–21
Zhang H (2004) Stigma and discrimination: the case of HIV/AIDS in China [Master's thesis, Tsinghua University]. CNKI. https://kns.cnki.net/KCMS/detail/detail.aspx?dbname=CMFD0506&filename=2005035753.nh
Zhang X (2010) Institution change and its values foundation: China's AIDS problems in the view of constructivism [PhD thesis, Jilin University]. CNKI. https://kns.cnki.net/KCMS/detail/detail.aspx?dbname=CDFD0911&filename=2010107649.nh
Zhang X, Chow EPF, Jing J (2014) The conceptual definition of AIDS from a constructivist perspective. Natural Dialectics Lett (06):58–64+127

Chapter 3
Research Framework and Research Methodology

3.1 Research Framework and Research Ideas

3.1.1 Research Framework

The research framework of the study is shown in Fig. 3.1.

3.1.2 Research Approaches

The author has been studying AIDS since September 2004 and applying qualitative research as the main means of collecting information in view of the specificity of this group.

Firstly, literature review was conducted. The author searched and sifted through the present theoretical and empirical studies on subject construction and self-presentation of marginalised groups at home and abroad from platforms such as CNKI (China National Knowledge Infrastructure), the National Library of China and the China CDC.

Secondly, the semi-structured in-depth interviews were conducted. The interviewees consisted of two groups: PLWHA and non-infected people. Thirty people living with HIV/AIDS, introduced by the staff of some ASOs (AIDS Service Organisations), were interviewed in-depth using the snowball method. Non-infected people involved a total of nine government staff or clerks, teachers and medical workers and eight members of the general public. The study collected in-depth interview data from both groups and conducted a comparative study to gain insight into the views and opinions. of the two groups about the stigma of PLWHA. At the same time, focus group interviews were conducted three times throughout the research. Based on these findings, the author collected research data on the identity construction process of

X. Wang, *Destigmatisation of People Living with HIV/AIDS in China*, A Sociological View of AIDS, https://doi.org/10.1007/978-981-16-8534-7_3

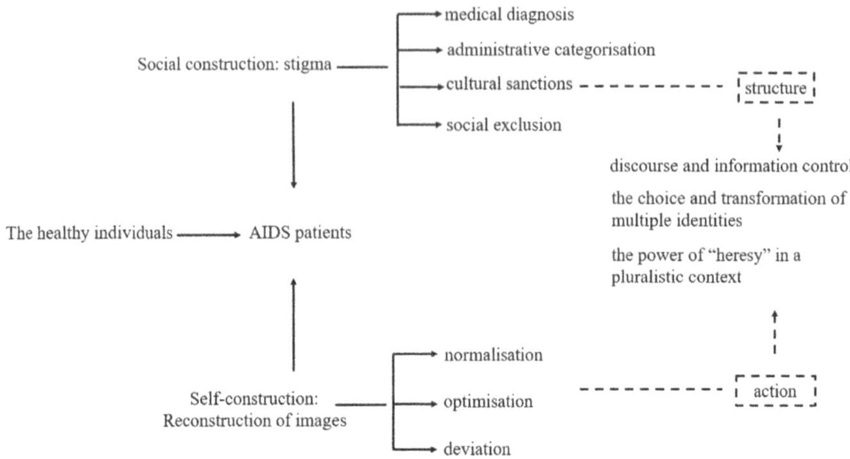

Fig. 3.1 Research framework of the study

PLWHA and information related to the self-construction and social construction of the interviewees.

Throughout the research, the author visited "Green Harbor" (established by Linfen Infectious Diseases Hospital in China's Shanxi Province) and communicated with PLWHA every month from 2004 to 2012. Through field studies, the author grasped first-hand information on their behavioural patterns, their prospect of future lives, and the attitudes and perceptions of the general population towards them. Therefore, the book tries to ensure the credibility of the first-hand information obtained.

Thirdly, the data obtained were analysed in a comparative and analogous approach to explore the identity construction and heterogeneity of actions of PLWHA and to grasp the structural characteristics of their constructive actions. The mechanisms of their identity production in real life were thoroughly analysed and discussed, facilitating the understanding of the relationship and operational mechanisms between the social construction of identity, self-construction and "structural action" of PLWHA in real life. These will be presented in both direct and indirect statements, involving the interviewees' understanding and inherent perceptions of social events and their own actions, as well as relatively objective statements. Regardless, the information was inevitably influenced by their subjective preferences. The author holds that both direct and indirect statements allow for the synthesis of information from multiple sources, avoiding omissions and subjective preferences of non-infected people and PLWHA to some extent and ultimately achieving the optimal analysis.

3.2 Research Methods

In the social sciences, there are two different research methods: quantitative and qualitative methods. Quantitative research, philosophically based on positivism, identifies correlations and causal relationships between things through experiments and surveys and explores related social phenomena based on research hypotheses, which can be said to be its basic feature.

In contrast, qualitative research, philosophically based on humanism, tends to apply participant observation and in-depth interviews to gain a deeper understanding of social phenomena. In the process of theory construction, the researcher himself is usually used as a research tool. In a given context, based on an in-depth interaction, the researcher generalises and elucidates the research subject.

In most cases, the optimal method is to combine quantitative and qualitative research methods. In view of the specificity of the identity of PLWHA, the book applied a qualitative research method and in-depth interviews. Trust was gradually established between PLWHA and the author through frequent visits of the treatment hospitals or organisations. Through face-to-face interactions with PLWHA, the author collected more information related to the research subject during the interviews, including even their body language and behaviour (e.g., sadness, joy, depression, anger).

3.2.1 Qualitative Research Method

There are usually two different levels of qualitative research: the basic one is to apply qualitative research with no quantitative analysis, and the conclusions obtained by this method are typically highly generalised and have a strong philosophical sense of theoretical thinking; the advanced one is qualitative research based on quantitative analysis. In the actual research process, qualitative research and quantitative research methods are used simultaneously. Before conducting quantitative research, researchers usually need to use qualitative research methods to determine the nature of the research subject or the particular phenomenon to be studied. In addition, the quantitative boundaries or factors that cause qualitative changes in a particular subject or particular social phenomenon can be determined.

Participant observation, one of the methods often used by researchers in qualitative research, and in-depth interviews are applied to obtain first-hand information. It is important to clarify that the strengths of participant observation lie in that it observes not only the discrimination and stigma of PLWHA but also the reasons, attitudes, procedures and rationale for people's actions in the process and that it enables the researcher to obtain subjective feelings in a particular situation, thus contributing to a more comprehensive understanding of the significance of social actions of the observed. Finally, by processing the first-hand information obtained through the participant observation method and in-depth interviews, the researcher is able to transform the initially fragmented and illogical information into concepts and principles of social scientific significance, which can provide a solid basis for theorisation.

3.2.2 Literature Review

A literature review is the foundation and prerequisite for all social research. Through a literature review, the researcher can understand the relevant theories, methods, policies and current research results and views on the research topic to determine the theme and direction of the research. During the research of this book, websites on AIDS-related issues were reviewed to fully understand the status quo of international and domestic AIDS infection, treatment and epidemic trends, to prepare for the selection of the topic; secondly, the author sorted out the current situation of AIDS research at home and abroad, as well as theoretical studies on social adaptation; thirdly, on the basis of the above research, the author summarised the theories related to social psychology and social capital, and finally determined research framework.

The study was conducted over a long period of time. During the interviews with PLWHA from 2004 to 2009, it was found that their initial psychological situation, attitudes and behaviours, as well as their treatment of the disease and their attitudes and behaviours towards the general public around them, are reconstructed and undergo qualitative changes with the passage of time and with the accumulation of their social experiences, which makes the author combine the initial and updated information to analyse and explore the implicit reasons.

3.2.3 Interview (Survey) Method

The interview method is a method in which the researcher interviews and talks to the selected interviewees to collect information in accordance with the requirements of the survey plan and the survey outline, including the structured interview method and the unstructured interview (or in-depth interview) method. Unstructured interviews are not based on pre-designed questionnaires and fixed procedures but have only a topic or outline for the interview, and the interviewer (sometimes the researcher is also the interviewer) and the respondent talk more freely around the established topic or outline. There is relatively little qualitative research on HIV stigma and less use of methods such as in-depth interviews and participant observation to obtain first-hand information on the stigmatisation of PLWHA. However, HIV stigmatisation is influenced by a variety of social, political, economic and cultural factors. To gain a deeper understanding of HIV stigmatisation, in-depth interviews and participant observation are needed to explore the living conditions and survival of PLWHA in specific social contexts and the context of real-life situations and to explore the underlying perceptions and factors.

The author re-conducted unstructured interviews with thirty HIV-infected people to collect information on their current social attunement. The interviewees (infected and non-infected) are numbered in sequence, and to protect their privacy, only the number is indicated in brackets quoting the infected person's statement. The respondents were selected from those who had been identified through personal connections and a snowballing way between 2009 and 2010.

The interview process also applied an observation method, which helped to eliminate some misunderstandings or interference with the information obtained during verbal or interpersonal communication. The author went deep into the lives of PLWHA of the "Green Harbour" and observed their environment, living conditions and standard of living at close range, as well as their expressions, mannerisms and body language, etc. These concerns are particularly important in the study of the identity of PLWHA, especially in the study of the perceptions and feelings of their self-identity, and the observation method has shown its strengths, providing a guarantee of accuracy in future research and analysis.

3.3 Research Ethics

As research on PLWHA involves personal privacy and confidentiality, the author is very cautious about defending their rights. The interviewees included both infected and non-infected people from different positions and status, ranging from government officials (people from civil affairs departments) to ordinary people (e.g., those who sell blood due to poverty) and from mainstream people to marginalised people (homosexuals, drug abusers). In the past ten years, since 2004, the author has consulted and interviewed some officials of relevant projects, held high-level forums on AIDS stigma, participated in activities of grassroots organisations (e.g., donating to Red Ribbon schools, organising student performances, etc.), attended academic conferences related to AIDS in China. To grasp first-hand information, the author has come into contact with people infected through blood transfusion, sex behaviours, drug-taking, etc., with gay men and lesbians (introduced by the CDC and some grassroots organisations) and with sex service providers (by going to detention centres to conduct interviews). During the research, some ethical issues were involved, such as the confidentiality of the information. When the author consulted relevant information at the CDC, the person in charge specifically stressed that some data must not be disclosed, e.g., the personal information of the interviewees, especially that of the infected people. To protect their rights and interests, all of these issues were treated with great consideration.

3.3.1 Principles of Research Resources (Data) Protection

To protect the privacy and other rights of the interviewees (infected and non-infected people) and to comply with academic norms and research ethics (confidentiality particularly indicated in some articles), the information quoted in the book is collected from public reports or literature that can be available publicly (e.g., the number of HIV-infected people in a certain province or region). The interviews and materials that had to be quoted were also in compliance with principles of confidentiality.

3.3.2 Privacy and Confidentiality in Research

The research issue of this book is AIDS, which, compared with social science research on other issues, is characterised by privacy, sensitivity and subjectivity, and it is difficult to obtain a comprehensive and accurate delineation of the actual situation of PLWHA using quantitative research methods. PLWHA are quite reluctant to talk about their past life experiences. Therefore, in the survey, trust needs to be built first, which functions importantly in the development and advancement of the research. How to build trust? Long-term in-depth contact with the interviewees is required. For example, the author found that it was almost difficult to conduct in-depth interviews with infected people at the first meetings. Even if accompanied by a community-in-charge, the author was only a stranger in their eyes and unable to earn their trust. They were reluctant to share their experiences until a good trusting relationship was built. In other words, it takes a long period of time to erase their psychological anxiety and vigilance.

The ethical principle of "informed consent" was strictly applied in all interviews, and each interviewee was first briefed on the content of the interview and given promise of strict confidentiality.

Chapter 4
Mechanisms of Stigmatisation of People Living with HIV/AIDS in China

The formation of stigma is a dynamic process of social construction (Guan 2007), and the mechanisms of stigmatisation of PLWHA are the result of a complex and multifaceted combination of actions. This chapter first describes and analyses the manifestations of HIV stigma in the mental, working, medical care, schooling and other areas, showing a concrete picture of HIV stigma. Then, the mechanisms of stigmatisation of PLWHA in China are explained at the individual, group, and social levels, respectively. Finally, we analyse the development process of the intersection of HIV stigma and identity stigma among PLWHA, focusing on the interaction between the stigmatisation of PLWHA and high-risk groups of AIDS.

4.1 Manifestations of Stigmatisation of People Living with HIV/AIDS in China

AIDS is often associated with undesirable stereotypes, such as filth, promiscuity, and terror. Associated with AIDS is a variety of social discrimination against and rejection of PLWHA, mainly in the mental, working, medical care, employment, and other areas.

According to a Chinese scholar Liu Neng, discrimination against PLWHA is mainly manifested in social interactions at the individual level (e.g., deliberate maintenance of spatial distance and deliberate avoidance of direct physical contact) and food-related social activities (e.g., reluctance to eat with them at the same table), thus maintaining a state of isolation and exclusion of PLWHA who have a compromised identity (Liu 2005). *The 2014 Report on the Progress of AIDS Prevention and Control in China*, published by the National Health and Family Planning Commission (now the National Health Commission), notes that PLWHA continue to suffer from social discrimination in medical care, employment, and schooling in China.

X. Wang, *Destigmatisation of People Living with HIV/AIDS in China*, A Sociological View of AIDS, https://doi.org/10.1007/978-981-16-8534-7_4

4.1.1 Mental Area: Moral Degeneration

HIV infection is largely attributed to the lack of morality in China. For a long time, most people have regarded AIDS as an immoral disease and categorised PLWHA as morally bankrupt in that they believe that HIV infection is the result of doing something immoral, which deserves retribution. Thus, PLWHA are often considered "bad", morally bankrupt and promiscuous.

> There are hundreds of workers in our factory. After they knew I had the disease, it was rumoured that I was infected with AIDS because I had sex with others illegally. I have worked in the workplace for so many years and won an award for "Advanced Individual". I've never had promiscuous relationships with others. However, when they heard of that, they spread the rumors. At first, I felt depressed because I had such a dirty disease. How do they look on me? Now I don't care. Even my family members living in the compound are often picked on. Life is not easy for us. (Infected Case No. 10)
>
> People who do not care for their own bodies or cherish their own reputation will develop AIDS. Will those who abide by the law and behave themselves get AIDS? It's those working as whores and those going whoring who get AIDS. (Non-infected Case No. 3)
>
> AIDS is a disease that cannot be easily infected, unlike flu or fever, which can infect each of us. Honest people can't get it in their whole life. Those who are not honest do not want to work to get rich, or go whoring with the money they earn, or take drugs. People who do not have AIDS will develop other diseases sooner or later. Some with the disease get others into trouble by infecting them. Anyway, decent people can't get it. (Non-infected Case No. 6)

4.1.2 Working Area: Employment Discrimination

Discrimination against PLWHA in the workplace is a common phenomenon. Often, when HIV infection is known by their colleagues, they will find it difficult to continue staying at the same job, or even lose their jobs. They will have to suffer from financial and emotional stress from discrimination in the workplace.

They are generally discriminated against in the workplace by having their job applications rejected, their current jobs terminated, and their jobs passively quitted, which makes it difficult for them to obtain appropriate wages and income. The high medical and medication costs resulting from HIV infection make them financially embarrassed and compromised in their quality of life.

> The first time I was diagnosed positive of the disease, I wanted to hide it for fear that others should think something serious was wrong with me. Later, when I had the tests and underwent the treatment, the news of infecting AIDS was like breaking news coming out from the hospital. When the leader knew that, he suggested that I go home to rest and not go to work, just receiving a basic salary. Some people went to talk with the leader and said they could not do this job anymore because they had to touch this and that every day and weren't sure when they would get infected. They asked the leader to send me home. I know they were afraid of being infected. Even if they know they cannot be infected directly, it doesn't feel good to be like this every day. So sometimes I truly want to quit, but it costs much money to take medicine and see a doctor, and I can't stay at home without salary. I just stay at home with the basic salary. I also want to look for other jobs, but I'm afraid of being scolded if I

don't tell anyone about the disease and of infecting others. I don't expect to work again. I am content with the money that I could use to see a doctor and take medicine. I won't go out to disgust others. (Infected Case No. 11)

If one of my colleagues is infected with AIDS, I'm sure I'm afraid. I will try to avoid it. If I can't, I'll change my job. It's not good to be afraid every day. I'm not discriminating against AIDS, but the medical research on it is not intensive enough. According to the report on the TV program, daily contact is not contagious, but if you accidentally cut your finger or something, you might be infected. (Non-infected Case No. 45)

4.1.3 Medical Care: Discrimination in Access to Medical Care

PLWHA have to go to hospital more often because they are vulnerable to infection due to HIV attacks or the compromised immune system. However, there is discrimination against them among medical staff, which is mainly caused by the fear of being infected. This can be shown in what one doctor from Linfen Infectious Diseases Hospital in Shanxi Province of China stated.

I have been in contact with the infected people since 2004, and all of them are in the advanced stages of infection. So sometimes I worry that I am infected too, and want to check if I'm HIV negative. If I had been negative for so many years, it would mean that HIV itself was not as scary as I thought. It was not until 2012 that I started to check if I was infected. (Non-infected Case No. 48)

As medical work itself is a high-risk profession, frequent exposed to various viruses and bacteria, medical workers have a strong sense of protecting themselves against HIV infection.

The doctors in large hospitals were more professional, and it seemed that they consciously kept the distance from me and did not say much. They just did what they needed to do. However, the doctors in our small place were not so good and would find all sorts of excuses not to treat me. (Infected Case No. 16)

When I was diagnosed with AIDS, I asked the doctor if it could be cured. The doctor said AIDS was a global problem, which was even beyond the ability of the United States. So we could only take medicine to control it. I asked him how long I could live. He said, "Go back and look it up on the internet", and didn't want to talk to me anymore. (Infected Case No. 19)

Whenever I went to the hospital, I had a hard time. The doctors and nurses were indifferent and wanted to send you away quickly. I didn't want to go to the hospital, but I had to. These doctors and nurses paid by the government didn't treat me like a patient. (Infected Case No. 14)

Sometimes when I was not well and wanted to be hospitalised, the hospital didn't admit me. At first, they said there were no more wards available and I had to get a private one, but there were no private ones for me. Then, they said they wouldn't have admitted any other patients if they admitted me, so they just gave me some medications to take at home. (Infected Case No. 17)

Dr. Ma from Linfen Infectious Diseases Hospital once treated a critically ill patient with AIDS. When a specialist consultation was urgently needed, there were no specialists available. In addition, when health care professionals help some patients to drain the pus, it may accidentally splash on their faces, which inadvertently puts pressure on them. Doctors who are more knowledgeable about AIDS than the general public also have discrimination against AIDS. Health care professionals and counsellors who come into contact with the infected people are sometimes compelled to act in a discriminatory manner due to the fear of being infected and mainly for the sake of the safety of their families.

4.1.4 Schooling: Social Exclusion and Rejection

Discrimination in schooling occurs mainly among children living with and affected by HIV/AIDS. China has established a system of free and compulsory education and financial support for students from families in need, and children affected by AIDS have the right to compulsory education. However, children living with and affected by HIV/AIDS are often treated differently in schooling. This differential treatment comes from schools and teachers, as well as peer groups.

Findings from case studies show that it is still common for children living with HIV/AIDS to be excluded from school and group activities by their schoolmates and other peer groups after they have been found to be infected with HIV.

> Because of me, my son had low self-esteem at school, became reluctant to talk and his academic performance dropped. He used to be in the middle to top of the class even though his grades were not the highest. Then, one day he came home particularly upset. When we asked him why, he said that the teacher had put him at a separate table, and his classmates became estranged from him. A good friend of his used to come to our house on weekends, and they would do their homework together and then play video games. I would wash some fruit for them. Then, after I took the medicine (publicly), his friend never came over again. My son has mentioned to me that he wants to transfer to a boarding school in the suburbs, but I think his school is a key one in the district, close to my home, which is better than the boarding school in the suburbs. Recently, I am thinking of transferring him to a boarding school if his academic performance continues to drop next semester. If so, he would not come home often because of the long distance, and the teachers and students there do not know about my case, which might be good for my child. (Infected Case No. 12)
>
> Both of my children are exceptionally bright and study quite well, and they now live with their grandparents. (Q: Don't they live with you?) No, they've lived with their grandparents since they were little. Now that I have the disease, they are still living at their grandparents' house, which is not far away. Their grandfather does not let them return for fear that others should gossip about them and other students at school should bully them. The elder child was honest and did not talk much, while the younger one was bad-tempered and often fought with others. I was so angry that I planned to go to the school to ask their teachers what the problem was, but neither of them would allow me to. (Infected Case No. 23)

In addition, there was a heated debate online over whether to disclose the identities of the senior high school students of the Linfen Red Ribbon School after they were enrolled at university in 2017. The majority of netizens believed that their identities should not be disclosed to protect their right to education, but a significant number of netizens opposed the idea, arguing that the rights of life and health of other university students would be difficult to protect if their identities were not disclosed.

4.1.5 Other Areas: Hidden Discrimination

Stigma and discrimination against PLWHA are manifested not only in the aforementioned four areas but also in other aspects of life. They are subtler because the discriminatory behaviours are not obvious or do not take shape on a large scale, making them difficult to attract widespread social attention. They manifest themselves in various subtle aspects of daily life, especially in the area of services, such as renting an apartment, haircutting, travelling and shopping, which bring much inconvenience to PLWHA. These ordinary acts of life may show discrimination against them, such as refusing to rent a room to them, to allow them to stay in the neighbourhood, to give them haircuts and to accept them to travel through a travel agency. These details of life are precisely the essential aspects of quality of life for them. If they are routinely discriminated against in these areas, it is difficult for them to have a good quality of life.

> I don't bother others, and I take care of everything myself. Now everyone in my neighbourhood knows I have AIDS. Even the vegetable sellers downstairs know about it, and they do not want to talk to me much when I go to buy vegetables. They do not even want to take the money, possibly due to the fear of being infected, but they could not stop selling to me. I also felt that I should not make things difficult for them, so I stop buying from them. I do not go to the retail department either, as they are not willing to receive me. So sometimes I have to go to a faraway market where no one knows me and the sellers are kind. I feel more comfortable and would buy more at a time. (Infected Case No. 1)
>
> If I knew the customer had AIDS, I would have found an excuse to send him away. After once or twice, he would have understood that and stopped coming. Even though I know it's probably not contagious, I'm still afraid. You know I have to cook and pick up my kids when I get home. You had better have some regard. I mean, we don't have AIDS here, and I can't tell who has it if any, so I truly need to wash my hands often (laughing) (Non-infected Case No. 46)

Stigma and discrimination against PLWHA come from mental, working, medical care, employment and other areas, and the manifestations of discrimination and their feelings vary from one area to another. The impact of stigma on their lives can be seen through discrimination in each of these areas, as they suffer not only from physical pain but also from discrimination in all areas, and are subjected to great physical and mental stress.

4.2 Mechanisms of Stigmatisation of People Living with HIV/AIDS in China

4.2.1 Individual Level: Attribution Theory

Attribution theory is the most common theory used by social psychologists to explain the causes of stigma. Weiner proposed an attribution theory of stigma in their experiments, making a significant contribution to stigma research in the 1980s. Attribution theory focuses on the causes of disease and makes judgements about the stigma of disease from the perspective of causal controllability. From the perspective of the causation of illness, different attributions lead to different emotional responses to the illness, which in turn further influences the individual's attitude and behaviour towards the illness. Among the dimensions of attribution, controllability is the most important. The perception of controllability of behaviour is the basis for the individual's judgement of responsibility for HIV infection and is a major cause of stigmatised emotions and behaviours. If the cause of infection is beyond the control of the individual, that is, the individual cannot control a certain infectious behaviour, people will feel sympathy for him or her and offer further help to him or her, whereas if the individual can control the route of infection, people's emotional response to him or her is expressed as anger, in that they believe the individual has no control over his or her behaviour and should be held responsible for his or her behaviour, thus showing discrimination (Weiner et al. 1988).

4.2.1.1 Controllable Causation Generates Stigma

Specifically, in terms of the mechanisms of HIV stigma, it is generally believed that the causes of AIDS are under the control of the individual and that the individual can avoid contracting HIV by reducing or eliminating risky behaviours such as immoral sex, drug abuse and blood selling. In contrast, an individual with HIV who does not control his or her behaviour that leads to HIV infection is responsible for his or her own behaviour. This is why PLWHA, among people with infectious diseases, suffer from widespread, public and harsh stigmas. Research shows that respondents generally believe that HIV-infected behaviour can be controlled and PLWHA are responsible for their own actions, and this attribution leads to more stigmas being attached to them (Mak et al. 2006).

> Not everyone can get AIDS. Unlike cancer, it cannot be prevented. So stay away from people who are susceptible to the disease. (Non-infected Case No. 4)
>
> They have no one to blame but themselves for getting AIDS. They know those places are filthy, but still go there. No one would have dragged them there if they didn't go. Anyway, it's their own choice. Similarly, they wouldn't have got it if they didn't take drugs, or if they kept clean. After all, they have to blame themselves for this disease. If they took care of themselves, didn't go to messy places or make friends indiscriminately, they would have been fine. (Non-infected Case No. 47)

Some years ago, many villagers in Henan Province earned much money by selling blood. Knowing that, all villagers went to sell blood and got AIDS. If they hadn't gone to sell blood, they wouldn't have got it. To put it bluntly, they were lazy and didn't want to do some farm work. Later, selling blood was forbidden in our country. Who would work if they all went to sell blood for money? If you have AIDS, you've to be supported by the government, so it's right to forbid selling blood. (Non-infected Case No. 44)

4.2.1.2 Uncontrollable Causation Evokes Sympathy

According to attribution theory, if the causes of infection are beyond the control of the individual, he or she will receive more sympathy. Some people contract AIDS for reasons beyond their control, such as through blood transfusions in hospitals or through mother-to-child transmission. These reasons are uncontrollable, that is, not controlled by their own behaviour. It is the external factors that impose themselves on these individuals, who are more likely to receive sympathy from the public.

I was infected during a blood transfusion. Knowing that, some were quite sympathetic and supported me in my lawsuit against the hospital. (Infected Case No. 13)

Those children with AIDS are the most innocent of all. They were born with AIDS and have never had a good life. Alas! They will not live longer after contracting HIV. They need the government's support. If they stay at home, their parents who have AIDS cannot afford to feed or treat them. Poor souls. These innocent creatures should gain more attention from the government. (Non-infected Case No. 5)

Attribution theory has to some extent explained how stigma is formed and has been widely applied in stigma research, especially in clarifying the mechanisms of stigma from a psychological perspective. However, it has certain limitations to explain the mechanisms of HIV stigma from the perspective of attribution theory in that attribution theory does not take into account the effects of other factors such as the lethality of AIDS and the risk of infection on people's responses and behaviours towards them (Peters et al. 1994). Thus, research on HIV stigma should consider attribution as well as the effects of other factors.

We dare to talk about AIDS, but in the past we felt too embarrassed to. I remember a time when we cursed someone, we would say "May AIDS befall you, and die a good death." (Non-infected Case No. 42)

AIDS is a major problem for mankind. It would be a real blessing to mankind if someone were to overcome it. The problem is that there is no cure. If you have it, you are sentenced to death. (Non-infected Case No. 47)

No matter how I got this disease, I feel sick. I do not want to see anyone with AIDS for the rest of my life, and I don't think anyone around me will get it either. (Q: What would you do if one of your friends had AIDS?) I don't think we could be friends anymore, not even my best friend. It's likely to be infected. I truly feel sick. (Non-infected Case No. 8)

4.2.2 Group Level: Social Morality Theory

The formation of stigma against PLWHA occurs at the psychological level of individuals and the group level. Clues to the mechanisms of group-level stigmatisation of PLWHA can be found through the lens of sociocultural theory. Sociocultural theory developed by the famous psychologist Lev Semyonovich Vygotsky from the former Soviet Union focuses on the central role of sociocultural factors in the development of a wide range of cognitive functions in human beings in all their complexity. Yang et al. who developed a conceptual model of stigma argued that the reason one group has stigma to another lies in its response to a perceived threat from another group, the real danger that does exist in another group, and the fear of the unknown (Yang et al. 2008). It can be argued that the stigmatisation of one group by another is a self-protective psychological defence mechanism for the stigmatiser, which gradually rises to the moral level. On the other hand, stigmatisation confronts the stigmatised people not only with physical illness or impairment but also with social and psychological problems such as loss of social status and damage to their reputation.

In their study of stigma across cultures, Major and O'Brien define stigma as a cognitive adaptation that has developed over human evolution, whereby humans avoid the potential dangers of living in groups by excluding those with certain undesirable traits (Major and O'Brien 2005).

4.2.2.1 Self-Protective Defence Mechanisms of the Group

In terms of the group-level mechanism, the stigma against PLWHA is a self-protective psychological defence mechanism for social groups. The public stigmatises PLWHA because of the threat they feel from the AIDS community and their fear of the high infectivity of the disease. They exclude PLWHA from their own sphere of life or group for self-protection.

> Unlike pneumonia or mental illness, AIDS is an infectious disease. Quite frightening. If they don't say anything, we don't know who has AIDS. They seem to be fine, but this disease is not detected unless at an advanced stage. I think AIDS patients must be kept under control. We can't allow them to wander around. If they are diagnosed as positive, it is better to use intensive treatment. For example, we can build a hospital for them only. In this way, there would be no transmission. Neither the people inside or outside the hospital would be afraid. In addition, there would be no more discrimination. All the people inside are patients, so why is there discrimination? (Non-infected Case No. 3)
>
> If I knew someone had AIDS, I wouldn't go near them. What if I should be infected? So just stay away from them. (Non-infected Case No. 9)
>
> I've never thought about it. I've never heard of anyone around me having AIDS. If they had AIDS, I would be quite scared, scared of being infected. It might not be contagious, but I'm still a bit scared and uncomfortable. (Non-infected Case No. 46)

4.2.2.2 Moral Level

Another feature of the group-level mechanism of stigmatisation of PLWHA is the elevation of stigma to a moral level, creating a strong sense of 'shame' due to the loss of honour and reputation and spreading this sense of stigma to their family members or social networks.

> A man of honour does not usually develop AIDS, but those with a promiscuous lifestyle are more likely to develop it. It's a kind of punishment. You can't go to places like that. If it weren't for the fear of getting this disease or that, more people would go there. (Non-infected Case No. 43)
>
> Unlike those people, how can we, ordinary, decent and hard-working people, get this disease? (Non-infected Case No. 41)
>
> I don't know what AIDS is, but I'm sure I won't get it. I just go to work, go home to take care of my kids and cook every day. How can I get this disease? If those people had a decent job and took good care of their families, I think no one would have had this disease. (Non-infected Case No. 46)

4.2.2.3 Institutional Level: Sociocultural Theory

While attribution theory and social morality theory have explained the mechanisms of stigma among PLWHA at the individual and group levels, respectively, how such stigma is formed at the institutional level can be explained based on sociocultural theory. Parker et al. developed the conceptual framework of stigma at the social institutional level from a sociocultural perspective, arguing that previous studies have not clearly defined the concept of stigma or even completely deviated from Erving Goffman's classic definition of stigma (Parker et al. 2003). Other scholars have argued that stigma should essentially be a social attribute that lowers the social status of individuals by formulating and establishing various social rules in order to enhance the interests of the dominant group and create hierarchy and social order. In this process, hierarchy or hierarchical order is further legitimised by means of institutionalisation (Liu and Shi 2010). Drawing on philosophical and sociological studies of power and social culture, Parker argues that stigma is not an isolated social phenomenon, but is linked to culture, power and difference. In the final analysis, the formation of stigma is inextricably linked to the inequality of social structures. The stigmatisation of others is part of the complex power struggle in social life, a process whereby dominant people pursue power, status and the corresponding social resources by making regulations or using strong-arm tactics. After gaining absolute dominance, they legitimise their long-term absolute dominance by solidifying the unequal social structure and continue to stigmatise others.

The infection of most PLWHA subject to social exclusion and discrimination is related to their socio-economic status, poverty and unfortunate life experiences. The majority of them are sex workers, drug abusers, blood sellers and other groups at the bottom of society. One of the most important reasons for them to engage in blood selling, drug abuse or sex trafficking is economic poverty or homelessness. Social inequality deprives them of social resources. To obtain the corresponding social resources, they use the only resources they have to engage in sex trade, blood selling and other activities and are stigmatised and discriminated against. After infection with HIV, they will be further stigmatised and deprived of more social resources, which creates a vicious cycle of inequality.

> When I was young I knew our family was poor. Our family was given approximately 0.2 acres of land, and my parents raised seven children. At that time, I was serving my younger siblings, and wasn't allowed to go to school... After having children, I had to go out to work because my husband was useless and lazy... Later, a friend of mine introduced a "procuress" to me. It's been fine, and I know well of the protective measures. I had planned to do this for a couple of years for some money before going home to build the house, and then to quit. Later, I felt that something was wrong with my body, so I went for a check-up and was diagnosed positive. (Infected Case No. 18)
>
> I come from a rich family. When I was in primary school I had a yuan a day for pocket money, so I was a big spender (laughing happily). Some of my classmates usually followed me into the retail department after school. (Q: How did you get so much pocket money?) My parents were earning money out, so I lived with my grandmother. (Q: Did your grandmother discipline you?) She couldn't discipline me. When I got to high school my parents could not discipline me either, so they gave up on me. I couldn't be a good student anyway, so I just hung out with my buddies. (Infected Case No. 30)
>
> I did this (sex work) to make money, but I didn't make much money and nearly got killed. My life is over. I haven't had any good things or enjoyed any blessings. (Infected Case No. 31)

4.3 Interaction of AIDS Stigma and Identity Stigma

The stigma of HIV has never been an isolated social phenomenon, but the stigma of PLWHA interacts with the stigma of their identity. Vulnerable groups have become a priority for HIV prevention. On the one hand, they are vulnerable to HIV infection for various reasons; on the other hand, their behaviour runs counter to the morality that society preaches, and the social stereotype of these groups makes HIV another symbol for them. To clarify the stigmas attached to several groups that are often associated with PLWHA, we will focus on foreigners, female prostitutes, male homosexuals, drug abusers and paid blood sellers.

4.3.1 Foreigners

AIDS was first discovered in Western countries, and the first case of AIDS in China was found in an American person. Therefore, in China, it was regarded as a disease unique to capitalist countries, and almost all foreigners were treated as AIDS-infected people. There was a tendency to equate "foreigners" with "AIDS patients" and even to refuse contact with them. According to reports at the time, restaurants, hotels and tour guides were most afraid of meeting foreigners coming to China, and some even refused to serve them for fear of contracting AIDS. There was a widespread social stigma and rejection of them. This reflected, on the one hand, the prevailing social perception that AIDS was an imported product only brought into China by foreigners. Thus, AIDS was regarded as a "fly", which should be swatted out. On the other hand, it reflected a lack of understanding of AIDS in society and a clear and definite understanding of its transmission routes. The belief that one could contract AIDS by touching objects used by foreigners reflected a lack of understanding of AIDS at that time, creating fear of the disease.

> I thought only foreigners would get the disease before. In addition, we had no contact with them so we could not have been infected. (Infected Case No. 25)
>
> Many foreigners have AIDS because they have an open attitude towards sex, and one foreigner may have several sexual partners. (Non-infected Case No. 1)
>
> I know the boss of one friend of mine has AIDS who is American and lives promiscuously in Beijing. I do not like foreigners, and the sight of a golden hair makes me sick. (Non-infected Case No. 8)

The stigma against foreigners gradually diminishes with the country's efforts to raise awareness of the disease and its transmission routes. Many people have a clearer understanding of how HIV is transmitted and believe that it cannot be transmitted through physical contact or droplets. In fact, with the support of good medical and health services, HIV infection in Western countries has been well controlled, but the situation in poor and backward areas of Africa is still not satisfactory. According to an article published in the February issue of *Discover* magazine, the HIV infection rate on the African continent is ten times that of the United States, and Uganda has the highest infection rate in the world. The stigma against foreigners slowly shifts to black Africans.

> It seems that more black people are getting AIDS these days, especially in underdeveloped Africa with poor sanitary conditions. The number of white people with AIDS in the U.S. seems to be decreasing, but that in Asia is lower. (Non-infected Case No. 4)

The stigma attached to foreigners with HIV stems more from cultural differences. Different ethnic groups often have different attitudes towards other ethnic groups due to their cultural characteristics, especially in terms of HIV stigma. The appearance and behaviour of foreigners are very different from those of the Chinese, which may be a major factor for the Chinese to reject and resent them. Therefore, the stigma attached to them is not just about the disease itself but also about culture.

4.3.2 Female Prostitutes

Female prostitutes, part of clandestine and illegal sex workers, are a key target in China's HIV prevention and control efforts. The specificity of their lives confronts them with a higher risk of contracting sexually transmitted diseases (STDs) and AIDS.

With the widespread HIV prevention and control efforts, China has been targeting female prostitutes, who are vulnerable to HIV infection through sexual intercourse. The probability of HIV infection among them has been reduced through widespread publicity of condom use, regular health check-ups, etc. Nevertheless, they are still closely associated with the stigmatisation of PLWHA. Sex workers are always connected with AIDS, and even they are often equated with people infected with STDs and AIDS. On the other hand, sex workers, one of the groups that develop AIDS, are stigmatised. The interaction between the stigmatised groups of sex workers and PLWHA has contributed to HIV stigma in society.

> Almost all the whores have STDs and will develop AIDS in severe cases. They would have sex with anyone if paid. All of them with STDs will slowly have AIDS. AIDS spread by them cannot be cured. After having AIDS, they still receive customers, infecting them all. Then, these customers return and infect their wives, or they look for other whores and infect them. No one can tell how many people are infected in this way. I think we need to keep an eye on these people and have a few more crackdowns. I do not believe we cannot control it. (Non-infected Case No. 7)
>
> Others think that I got infected by whores. If so, I would have accepted it. However, it is not true. Others would think you've got the filthy disease from someone who has that disease (Infected Case No. 24)

4.3.3 Male Homosexuals

When the first five cases of AIDS were found in gay men, AIDS was thought to be a disease only for homosexuals and to be a punishment from God for homosexuals from the perspective of religion (Zhang 2013). Then, cases of HIV infection through blood transfusions and mother-to-child transmission were discovered (Masur et al. 1981). Nevertheless, the notion that homosexuals are more susceptible to AIDS has always existed.

In 1989, when the first local case of AIDS was discovered in China, news reports attributed the infection to homosexual sex. HIV originates from sex or sexual promiscuity. The focus was shifted from foreigners to homosexuals, especially gay men.

The 2014 Report on the Progress of AIDS Prevention and Control in China states that the major transmission route of the AIDS epidemic in China is sexual transmission, and there is a marked increase in sexual transmission among men who have sex with men (MSM). MSM are considered to be the main transmitters of HIV. Moreover, a low percentage of them use condoms during sexual intercourse and thus have a higher risk of cross-infection.

Currently, people tend to view male homosexuals as a high-risk group for HIV. The stigma attached to male-to-male sexual transmission of HIV is compounded by the fact that homosexuals are themselves discriminated against.

> A lot of gay men have HIV because of their inadequate protective measures. Now, heterosexuals use condoms. I'm not sure whether gay men would use condoms. (Non-infected Case No. 2)

It is popular to be gay these days. It's a bad trend, and it is leading the youth astray. Those young and ignorant people, who like to try new things and lack common sense, are most vulnerable to AIDS. (Non-infected Case No. 6)

4.3.4 *Drug Abusers*

Drug abusers are also a key target for HIV prevention and control. A survey has shown that negative attitudes towards intravenous drug use contribute to social stigma and discrimination against PLWHA (Zhang, 2004). Intravenous drug users are themselves discriminated against for their behaviour. As the number of cases of HIV infection through intravenous drug use increases, there is a growing awareness of its vulnerability to HIV infection and a tendency to treat drug abusers as a potential population for HIV infection, creating multiple stigmas against HIV.

Intravenous drug users are prone to HIV infection, right? During drug addiction, several people share a needle to inject drugs. However, during the process, it is not sterilised, so it is definitely likely to become infected. I'm not sure whether use of other drugs would lead to infection. (Non-infected Case No. 42)

Drug addiction itself is quite harmful. If you got hooked, you couldn't quit, and if you got AIDS, there would be no cure. Those who take drugs would be either "gone" or have AIDS so that they wouldn't live long. It is right for the government to control drug use, cos it's not good for the country or the individual. (Non-infected Case No. 43)

4.3.5 *Paid Blood Sellers*

After the mass infection of HIV caused by blood selling in Henan Province in the late 1990s, blood sellers in Henan were regarded as the main group for HIV infection and transmission for a long time, creating HIV stigma among paid blood sellers there.

Those who sell blood have AIDS. They earn money quickly by selling blood. After obtaining a tube of blood drawn and resting for a few days, they continue to sell blood for money. (Non-infected Case No. 47)

There may be some blood sellers, but I guess there are fewer. Because of the policy, they stop selling blood and begin to donate blood for free. Now, they are not so poor as to sell blood. (Non-infected Case No. 9)

The most abominable thing is the illegal sale of blood. It seems that there are still some underground illegal blood stations where the poor sanitary conditions are likely to breed AIDS. These people infect others with AIDS by selling blood, which is abominable. Whoever is infected in this way is unlucky. We must crack down on this thoroughly. Otherwise, the infected patients would be too innocent. (Non-infected Case No. 1)

Based on the judgement that the AIDS epidemic in China still strikes the so-called "high-risk groups", the AIDS sentinel surveillance system launched in 1995 is an institutionalised system to track changes in the AIDS epidemic using sentinel sampling. It involves testing the interviewees for HIV and monitoring the behaviour of a subset of people to examine the link between routes of infection and their behaviour. Sentinel testing is the best way to help us understand the HIV epidemic in China and includes six key populations: clandestine prostitutes, drug abusers, gay men, truck drivers who are considered clients of prostitutes, HIV-vulnerable STD patients and pregnant women. Additionally, the HIV prevention and control strategy in China calls for a significant investment in education and behavioural interventions for high-risk populations.

4.4 Summary

The formation of stigma against PLWHA is a complex and multi-faceted combination of actions. This chapter provides a systematic discussion of the mechanisms by which HIV stigma is formed.

Firstly, the stigma and discrimination experienced by PLWHA are described in the mental, working, medical care, schooling and other areas. The study found that stigma manifests itself in moral degradation, employment discrimination, refusal of doctors to treat or indifferent treatment, isolation and rejection of students living with HIV/AIDS by schools, teachers and peer groups, and a complex and diverse range of discriminatory behaviours in these areas.

Then, after identifying the various manifestations of HIV stigma, the mechanisms of HIV stigma in China are explained at the individual, group and social levels and are the result of the intertwined and combined effects between the three.

The individual-level mechanism of stigmatisation of PLWHA is based on attribution theory from the social psychology perspective, which focuses on "controllability" and divides the causes of HIV infection into "controllable" and "uncontrollable". The controllable causes of HIV infection usually bring stigma and discrimination to them, such as those infected with HIV through sexual misconduct and drug abuse, while the uncontrollable causes bring sympathy to them, such as those infected with HIV through blood transfusion and babies infected with HIV through mother-to-child transmission, who will gain more sympathy from the public.

The group-level stigmatisation of PLWHA is a self-protective and psychological defence mechanism for the social group. The public stigmatises PLWHA because they feel threatened by the HIV community and fearful of the high infectivity of HIV. They exclude PLWHA from their own sphere of life or group for self-protection. In addition, the group-level mechanism raises stigma to a moral level.

The social-level mechanism of stigma against PLWHA is based on social morality theory. Stigma and discrimination should be understood not only at the individual and group levels but also as a sociocultural phenomenon linked to the human community as a whole. Stigma is not an isolated social phenomenon but is tied to culture, power and difference and is ultimately linked to unequal social structures. The infected people are generally subject to social exclusion and discrimination, most of whom become infected because of their low socio-economic status, poverty and unfortunate life experiences, and are stigmatised and discriminated against for engaging in high-risk activities. After infection, they are further stigmatised and deprived of more social resources, which creates a vicious cycle of inequality.

The stigma of HIV-vulnerable groups, such as clandestine prostitutes, male homosexuals, injecting drug users and paid blood sellers, has been tied to the key targets of HIV prevention and control in China since its inception and is still inseparable from that of PLWHA.

References

Guan J (2007) Stigma research: an interactive perspective based on sociology and psychology. Jianghuai Tribune 5:110–115

Liu N (2005) HIV/AIDS, stigma, and social discrimination: a quantitative analysis of AIDS patients and ordinary villagers in two Chinese rural communities. Sociol Study 6:136–164

Liu Y, Shi K (2010) Mechanism, negative effect and interventions of HIV stigma. Adv Psychol Sci 18(1):123–131

Major B, O'Brien LT (2005) The social psychology of stigma. Annu Rev Psychol 56:393–421

Mak WWS, Mo PKH, Cheung RYM et al (2006) Comparative stigma of HIV/AIDS, SARS, and Tuberculosis in Hong Kong. Soc Sci Med 63(7):1912–1922

Masur H, Michelis MA, Greene JB et al (1981) An outbreak of community-acquired pneumocystis carinii pneumonia: initial manifestation of cellular immune dysfunction. N Engl J Med 305:1431–1438

Parker R, Aggleton P (2003) HIV and AIDS-related stigma and discrimination: a conceptual framework and implications for action. Soc Sci Med 57:13–24

Peters L, den Boer DJ, Kok G et al (1994) Public reactions towards people with AIDS: an attributional analysis. Patient Educ Couns 24(3):323–335

Weiner B, Perry RP, Magnusson J (1988) An attributional analysis of reactions to stigmas. J Pers Soc Psychol 55(5):738–748

Yang LH, Kleinman A (2008) 'Face' and the embodiment of stigma in China: the cases of Schizophrenia and AIDS. Soc Sci Med 67(3):398–408

Zhang H (2004) Stigma and discrimination: the case of HIV/AIDS in China. Tsinghua University

Zhang X (2013) Two-way construction of AIDS in China. Intellectual Property Publishing House

Chapter 5
Evolving Features of and New Changes in Stigmatisation of People Living with HIV/AIDS in China

AIDS, known in full as acquired immunodeficiency syndrome, is a medical condition among many. The stigmatisation of a disease is usually related to the source, degree of infection of the disease and the physical suffering of the infected people. AIDS is a heavily stigmatised disease due to its controllability, high infectivity and the great suffering experienced by PLWHA, who suffer from severe stigma. The analysis and interpretation of the evolving features and new changes in the stigmatisation of PLWHA can provide a more comprehensive and insightful grasp of the forms and changes of HIV stigma and further form a comprehensive understanding of HIV stigma.

In terms of the mechanisms of HIV stigma, social identity theory suggests that the key point of HIV stigma is the strong emotional perception of PLWHA by the general population, a perception associated with the pursuit of positive social identity by normal people, and that the process of stigmatisation involves two main stimuli, namely concepts (symbolic) and symptoms (instrumental). Herek classifies HIV stigma into two types: instrumental and symbolic, depending on the source of the stigma. Instrumental stigma stems from self-defence (the need for safety of life), such as fear of infection and inexplicable fear of and anxiety about symptoms of AIDS patients, while symbolic stigma is concerned with abstract values and emotions and is primarily a result of the public's moral judgement of AIDS. The study also found that symbolic stigma can be changed through persuasion and education, while instrumental stigma is not so easily changed (as fear of death makes the public prefer to reject the infected people) (Herek 1999).

In summary, social identity theory holds that HIV stigma consists of two components: instrumental stigma, which refers to the symptoms of PLWHA, and symbolic stigma, which refers to the concept of AIDS. The classification of HIV stigma by Herek, limited in its scope, provides us with a deeper understanding of AIDS stigma in symbolic and instrumental terms.

X. Wang, *Destigmatisation of People Living with HIV/AIDS in China*, A Sociological View of AIDS, https://doi.org/10.1007/978-981-16-8534-7_5

5.1 Evolution of Symbolic Stigma

Symbolic stigma is concerned with abstract values. For PLWHA, the evolution of symbolic stigma can be interpreted from two perspectives. Firstly, the evolution of symbolic stigma based on the concept of HIV can be described by interpreting the historical context and trends of HIV evolution in combination with the prevailing discourse. Secondly, stigmatised individuals or groups, mainly high-risk groups, such as drug abusers, homosexuals and sex workers, are discriminated against, which is the moral judgement manifested in the rejection and exclusion of PLWHA infected through drug abuse, sexual transmission and other routes of transmission. This discrimination is not based on the infection itself but rather on the public's association of the routes of infection with "depravity" and "perversion" in quality and behaviour.

Before 1986, when there were no news reports on the local transmission of AIDS in China, the public had always translated AIDS into "aizibing" (爱滋病), which literally refers to a disease bred from promiscuous sex. They believed that AIDS could only be spread through sexual transmission and attributed AIDS to immoral sexual behaviour. Later, the number of PLWHA in China increased, and the proportion of blood-borne and intravenous drug transmission increased significantly. The name was changed to "aizibing" (艾滋病) because the original translation was misleading and ignored other routes of transmission, and it has become the only standardised and common Chinese name.

The term "aizi" (艾滋) is a transliteration of AIDS, but common diseases with the suffix of "bing" (which means disease or illness) in the Chinese name, such as venereal diseases and mental illness, are usually stigmatised except for diseases directly related to body parts, such as stomach disease and cervical spine disease (Yao 2011). The evolution of the name of AIDS in China has gone through a process from "aizibing" (爱资病) to "aizibing" (爱滋病) and to "aizibing" (艾滋病), an evolution of the understanding and stigmatisation of AIDS.

5.1.1 AIDS with Political Stigma

The initial translation of AIDS had a strong political bias, which was closely linked to the onset and discovery of AIDS. Five cases of PLWHA were published in the Morbidity and Mortality Weekly Report on 5 June 1981, which was the world's first record of AIDS. AIDS was first discovered in the United States, a typical capitalist country. It was not until five years later, i.e., in 1986, that the first case of AIDS, an Argentinean American case, was discovered in China. The media in China regarded AIDS as "a fly from the capitalist world" (Pan et al. 2006) and translated it as "aizibing" (爱资病) with political overtones. The prevention of AIDS was based on combined measures of "preventing flies from entering" and "swatting flies out", highlighting it as a disease unique to the capitalist world, with obvious political stigmatisation.

It is not difficult to understand that the presence of AIDS was seen as a product of the decadent life and social system of Western capitalist countries during that period. At the early stages of reform and opening up, China had rapid economic growth and many social problems. There was widespread anti-capitalist sentiment among the public, who tended to disparage everything about capitalism. When AIDS was discovered in the West, mainly in the U.S., the public saw it as a disease unique to "decadent" capitalism, which was a kind of stigma against the West and "drew a clear line" with it. This showed that as a socialist country, China would not have AIDS, and even we would consider it a punishment for the rotten system and life of Western capitalism.

As a consequence, there was a lack of understanding and awareness of HIV and adequate prevention psychology and strategies of HIV. Once contracting HIV, they have a high tendency to reject others and cannot adopt effective coping strategies.

> I always felt that AIDS was far away from me, and it was a disease prevalent in other countries. I never thought it would happen to me one day. (Infected Case No. 15)

> I thought many foreigners had this disease (AIDS) because they had an open attitude towards sex and didn't take that (having sex) seriously. They felt free to do anything. (Non-infected Case No. 4)

> More foreigners got AIDS. It was introduced to China from other countries. There was no such disease in China, a traditional country. We've never heard of it in our country, never. (Non-infected Case No. 3)

5.1.2 AIDS with Sexual Stigma

The conceptual stigmatisation of AIDS changed with the confirmed diagnosis of the first case of AIDS in China in 1989, who was also infected with an STD. It was reported that this person had a promiscuous private life and had been sexually promiscuous for a long time, even engaging in homosexual acts with foreigners. The term AIDS was used to describe a person with a promiscuous lifestyle and was then changed to "aizibing" (爱滋病) (Yao and Wang 2014). It was believed that AIDS was seen as "a disease bred from promiscuous sex" and was mainly transmitted through sexual immorality. The logic of the development of AIDS was "moral decay - promiscuity - AIDS", the stigma of AIDS was manifested in moral stigma based on immoral sex, and the response to the spread of AIDS was to "crack down" on immoral people, especially those who had illicit sex, such as prostitutes and peddlers of pornography.

During that period, the publicity of the main routes of HIV infection focused on sexual immorality rather than other routes. The consequences are obvious. Many years later, the public still believes that sexual intercourse, especially illicit sex, is the main route of HIV infection. The ignorance of the existence of other routes of HIV transmission is detrimental to a comprehensive HIV response.

> I've heard of AIDS, a terrible disease. It's incurable. You could get it from unprotected sex. That's all that I know. (Non-infected Case No. 1)

> I know about AIDS. I hear it's possible to get AIDS by going whoring. The risk of going whoring is too high. Who knows which whore will infect you with the disease, right? We don't know how many clients they receive a day. They don't know whether the clients have the disease, and the clients don't know whether they have the disease. (Non-infected Case No. 2)

> Promiscuous people having casual sex all day long are most likely to develop AIDS. It is possible to obtain an STD or something and then AIDS if cross-infected. It's a horrible disease. The more sex you have, the more cross-infected you get. Some rich men who usually have mistresses deserve to develop AIDS. (Non-infected Case No. 3)

5.1.3 Destigmatised AIDS

Full understanding of the transmission routes of AIDS helps us destigmatise AIDS. One study found that people infected with AIDS through routes such as blood donation and transfusion unrelated to moral evaluations are more likely to gain sympathy and do not experience undue psychological stress, in which moral evaluations of the cause of the disease play a decisive role (Zhou 2007).

In the late 1990s, a large number of people became infected with HIV through blood transfusion due to blood sales in Henan Province. Consequently, the proportion of people infected with HIV increased, which became more widely known. The influence of the incident in Henan has been so great that it has attracted widespread attention from the international community. With the improvement of information, under the pressure of international public opinions and based on the need for HIV prevention and control through multiple channels, the term AIDS has changed from "aizibing" (爱滋病), which refers only to the sexual transmission route, to the more value-neutral "aizibing" (艾滋病), which achieves the conceptual or symbolic destigmatisation of AIDS.

In the late 1990s, the Chinese government stepped up its efforts to promote awareness of and knowledge about HIV and increased the public's understanding of the full spectrum of HIV. HIV is no longer transmitted only through sexual intercourse but through multiple routes of transmission, including sexual intercourse, blood transmission and mother-to-child transmission. The conceptual destigmatisation of the term "AIDS" and the widespread and intensive publicity of the disease have contributed significantly to the reduction of stigma and discrimination against PLWHA in daily life.

Moreover, the response to AIDS has been based on a strategy of prevention in the first place and integrating prevention with control. The prevention and control of AIDS has been strengthened through the introduction of multiple routes of HIV infection and targeted prevention and control of people involved.

> AIDS is horrible. It has been reported on the news that people can develop AIDS from selling blood. A few years ago, many people in Henan sold blood because they were poor, and were

infected with AIDS. Almost all the people in one village contracted HIV. Their newborn children were also infected. (Non-infected Case No. 5)

I've never thought I would get this disease (AIDS). So many people across the country are transfused with blood every day. Why was something wrong with me? I couldn't figure it out. Why was something wrong with the blood in our hospital, a public one? Where did the blood come from? When I asked the hospital, they said it was from the blood station, and they had nothing to do with it. So I turned to the blood station, which in turn passed it on to the hospital.... I had to grin and bear it. (Infected Case No. 21)

We all know this, right? It's been shown on TV. There are several main ways of transmitting HIV: sexual intercourse, blood transmission, mother-to-child transmission and physical contact with mucosal damage. You'll be all right without mucosal damage. That's all. (Non-infected Case No. 46)

In brief, the stigma of AIDS in China has changed from politically stigmatised "aizibing" (爱资病) to sexually stigmatised "aizibing" (爱滋病) against sexual misconduct and to value-neutral "aizibing" (艾滋病) that has been destigmatised. It is evident that the symbolic stigma of AIDS has been eliminated in China. AIDS is no longer tied to a certain type of people or behaviour or no longer only involves moral condemnation but is just a name of one disease syndrome, such as stomach disease, cervical spondylosis, liver disease, and cancer.

5.2 Instrumental Stigma Characterised by Symptoms of People Living with HIV/AIDS

Although AIDS has been conceptually destigmatised in China, the stigma of the disease still exists in real life, largely due to the fear of transmission and the awareness of self-defence on the part of most people who deliberately distance themselves from people with AIDS.

Instrumental stigma stems from an individual's awareness of self-defence, and is usually a conscious discrimination and rejection based on concern for risks and resources. In terms of risks, it is mainly manifested in fear and rejection of symptoms of the disease due to fear of being infected with HIV, such as not shaking hands with PLWHA, not sharing public goods with them, refusing to come into contact with them, refusing to take care of their family members. In terms of resources, it is mainly manifested in discrimination against them in terms of schooling, medical care, employment, etc. For example, children with AIDS or children whose family members are infected with AIDS are discriminated against, rejected or even isolated by teachers, classmates and peer groups at school, which may lead to discontinuation of their schooling. Individuals are easily discriminated against by doctors, nurses and other medical personnel or even denied medical treatment; they are also easily discriminated against and isolated by colleagues and leaders in the workplace.

Instrumental stigma refers to the fear resulting from a lack of information about symptoms and transmission routes of the disease and a lack of knowledge about the infectious and lethal AIDS, which contributes to the stigma among PLWHA and their families. People treat them as bad people, often associating them with prostitution, drug abuse and promiscuity. People usually treat them and their families unfairly and differently in equal circumstances. This kind of discrimination, motivated by awareness of self-defence, is mainly intentional discrimination based on concern for risks and resources, for instance, in the denial of financial help to them.

The evolution of the instrumental stigma of AIDS is inextricably linked to that of the symbolic stigma in China. The instrumental stigma of PLWHA is acquired based on the symbolic stigma, but when the symbolic stigma is gradually reduced and eliminated, the instrumental stigma is not eliminated accordingly.

5.2.1 HIV Prevention Strategies: Scary Physical Symptoms to Manageable Physical Manifestations

During the first period of AIDS evolution in China, the publicity focused on highlighting the horrific, ugly and rotten physical symptoms of AIDS to deliberately degrade capitalism. Pictures, films and texts in mass media reports focused on vilifying the physical symptoms of PLWHA, highlighting their advanced symptoms and deliberately presenting the public with herpes, purple spots, blood blisters and petechiae on their skin and mucous membranes in the advanced stages of AIDS.

Since the discovery of HIV infections in China, there has been a terror strategy for AIDS prevention, attempting to create an atmosphere of terror by using negative publicity materials and to combat the spread of AIDS through terror education strategies. The negative publicity of AIDS has created an extreme fear of the disease in society and reinforced the instrumental stigma associated with fear of its symptoms.

> Knowing that I had the disease, I felt like my whole world had collapsed and that I was finished. All I could think of was that I would get blisters all over my body. Then, my whole body would become inflamed, smelly and rotten. At last, I would die a horrible death. (Infected Case No. 36)

> I've decided that I'm going to kill myself when it's too late to take the medication in the late stages. I'm sure I can't stand the pain, and it's hard for my family to see it. So I'll just wait and kill myself one day. I don't want to die a horrible death. I've got my cerements ready. I'm not so scared when I think about it. (Infected Case No. 22)

> I have seen pictures of AIDS patients on the internet, red bumps all over the tongue and all over the body, and the splitting skin. I got goose bumps when I saw those, and I never wanted to look at them again. Fortunately, I don't have it. Why is there such a torturous disease? Medical science is quite advanced, but there are still incurable diseases such as cancer and AIDS. (Non-infected Case No. 40)

> You can't live with AIDS. There's nothing good about your body, with pus and stinks. What's the point of living? It's just pain. It seems that AIDS patients don't live long either. We just don't know they develop the disease so rapidly. (Non-infected Case No. 46)

With the deepened understanding and research of AIDS, the medical profession and mass media have changed their publicity strategies from intimidating terror education to a more scientific and practical approach. For instance, PLWHA are often treated as ordinary people in reports, which makes the public recognise that they are not disgusting and are indistinguishable in appearance from ordinary people. Moreover, in the exploration of HIV prevention and control efforts, the medical profession has discovered drugs that have a controlling effect on HIV and can reduce symptoms of AIDS. Thus, AIDS is controllable for a certain period of time.

> Different from what it was in the past, AIDS can be controlled by medication. A famous Chinese actress called Zhang Ziyi played a person with AIDS in a film. She was no different from anyone else. You couldn't tell she had AIDS. She could still live for a long time, but it was too mentally torturing because there was no hope. (Non-infected Case No. 47)

> At first, I was very scared. I remember seeing pictures of people with AIDS. They were so thin, and I was so scared that I almost cracked up. Later, when I learned more about it, I was not so scared anymore, and it didn't look so bad. I just consider it a chronic disease requiring medication. I don't know what I would have been like if I didn't have this medicine. (Infected Case No. 34)

5.2.2 Medical Treatments: From Incurable to Manageable

It was thought that there was no cure for anyone contracting HIV, and AIDS was regarded as a "super cancer", more dangerous and deadly than ordinary cancer. Under such circumstances, PLWHA were seen as people with no hope of survival, and few people would provide care and support to them.

> After being diagnosed positive for HIV, I was very scared. I thought I would not live long because they said there was no cure for it. So I asked the doctor if I would die. The doctor said I would first have to take medication to control it, which would prolong my life for a few more years. It depended on my health conditions. Getting home, I looked it up in the book and determined that I couldn't die so easily. So I just let it go. (Infected Case No. 33)

> AIDS is a fatal disease. If you get it, you can't be cured or you won't live long. It's a world problem. Whoever develops a cure for AIDS will earn lots of money. That's why I say it can't be cured. It's hopeless if you have it. (Non-infected Case No. 4)

> If you have AIDS, you are waiting to die, so why treat it? There is no cure, and medicines can only relieve its symptoms. In fact, those doctors know that, so they prescribe some drugs to give the patients some psychological comfort. How can it be cured, especially in our small hospitals? It may be better in big cities, but I haven't heard of a cure for it. (Non-infected Case No. 9)

With the development of health care and publicity of AIDS in China, more people are aware that, first, AIDS has a certain incubation period; that is, even if HIV infection is detected, the disease does not occur immediately. Second, medication can be used to help PLWHA cope with HIV and prevent complications and deterioration of the disease, thus prolonging their survival.

Based on the basic notion that they are "saveable" and "survivable", there has been an increase in social sympathy and help for them and a decrease in the fear of AIDS among the public, who no longer associate AIDS with death. This helps to eliminate the public's fear of AIDS with a high mortality rate and thus reduces the stigma of AIDS.

> I treat it (AIDS) as a chronic disease, such as diabetes, which requires daily injection of insulin. I treat it as a chronic disease requiring medication every day. In the end it's all a matter of dying, sooner or later. We just need to take care of ourselves. (Infected Case No. 37)

> I thought that AIDS could not be cured, but it is not that terrible. Currently, medical technology is so advanced that AIDS will be conquered sooner or later. Even if you have it, you have to live well, and do whatever you need to do. I have one younger brother, only one, who has AIDS. I'll help him if I can. With more help, he may live a few more years; otherwise, what if he leaves his family? (Non-infected Case No. 42)

5.2.3 Routes of Transmission: From Physical Contact to Fixed Modes of Transmission

A major reason for the severe social stigma, discrimination and exclusion of PLWHA is the fear of HIV infection. In an era of limited understanding of the routes of transmission of AIDS, it was believed that AIDS could be transmitted by physical contact, even saliva droplets, air and breath. That was why people avoided them and were reluctant to have any contact with them. However, with the extensive publicity of knowledge of HIV prevention and control, the public has gradually become aware that there are only a few fixed modes of transmission of HIV, and one can avoid contracting it with adequate precautions, reducing the public's fear of its infectivity and the instrumental stigma of HIV.

Widespread publicity and education by the media have led to a deeper understanding of how HIV is transmitted and that ordinary physical contact and sharing of public objects do not transmit HIV. Nevertheless, instrumental stigma against PLWHA still exists and is difficult to eradicate.

> Shaking hands does not transmit HIV. Chinese President Xi Jinping even shook hands with an AIDS patient, so handshakes definitely do not transmit it. Some celebrities were photographed with AIDS patients and would hug children with AIDS, but none of them were infected. If they were infected, the celebrities would not have dared to hug those children. They must have learned about it in advance and knew it was okay. It seems that AIDS patients on TV are no different from us. (Non-infected Case No. 4)

> I know from the publicity on TV and from the community that living with an AIDS patient doesn't transmit HIV, but I'm still scared. Whenever I think of someone around me having AIDS, I feel like I will be infected sooner or later. I don't mean to discriminate against them, but we're all afraid of dying, right? (Non-infected Case No. 8)

5.2.4 Modes of Transmission: From Sexual-Only Transmission to Multiple Routes of Transmission

One of the most important reasons for the social stigma of PLWHA is related to the particular modes of infection. When AIDS was first introduced in China, sexual intercourse as one mode of transmission was prominently publicised. With the deepening understanding of AIDS, we focused on transmission via physical contact as well as prevention of blood-borne and mother-to-child transmission. The deepened knowledge of different modes of HIV transmission objectively eliminates the perception of HIV transmission through sex only and reduces the public's prejudice against AIDS in sexual morality, helping to reduce their condemnation of AIDS patients in sexual morality.

> It was thought that AIDS was a disease bred only from promiscuous sex. However, this is not the case. You can also get it from taking drugs, from selling blood, and so on. (Non-infected Case No. 2)

> It was believed that AIDS was only transmitted by sex, but now everyone knows you can get it from blood transfusion. Many families have been broken up because of HIV infection from blood transfusion. They went to the hospital for treatment but ended up contracting a more fatal disease. HIV infections from blood transfusion are medical malpractice, for which the hospital should hold responsibility. I'm truly too scared to go to the hospital now. I heard that some people who went to some small hospitals or clinics without sanitary conditions or thorough disinfection for dental treatment had AIDS. The wounds in the mouth from tooth extraction were still bleeding, which may transmit HIV. Therefore, don't go to a small hospital or clinic, but if you have to, go to a big one. (Non-infected Case No. 4)

5.2.5 Basic Argument: From "Blame-Oneself-Only Theory" to "Innocence Theory"

Initially, the public believed that PLWHA only had themselves to blame for their behaviour and that they were punished by God for the "bad things" they had done. With the publicity of HIV knowledge, the public gradually realised that there are also passive infections, such as mother-to-child transmission of HIV. Babies born with HIV in such a way are innocent and deserve sympathy. Some people contract HIV during blood transfusions when they are hospitalised due to illness, accidents, etc. When found to be infected with HIV with a certain incubation period, they are faced with difficulty in claiming their rights because several years have passed since the time of blood transfusion.

PLWHA no longer have only themselves to blame but are innocent. The change in the basic argument about them will help to gain sympathy and support of the public and eliminate the stigma against them.

> Children with AIDS are the most innocent of all. They were born with AIDS and never have a good life. Alas! They will not live longer after contracting HIV. They need the government's support. If they stay at home, their parents who have AIDS cannot afford to feed or treat

> them. Poor souls. These innocent creatures should gain more attention from the government. (Non-infected Case No. 4)

> I know there was an AIDS village in Henan, where almost all the children had AIDS. They were born with HIV. Those children coming from poor families may not grow up. Poor guys. It's no match for the children in the city. (Non-infected Case No. 5)

Symbolic stigma interacts with and evolves into instrumental stigma. They are correlated but distinct, with the former encompassing the latter and rejection and alienation out of a sense of self-defence.

Symbolic stigma provides the basis or tone for instrumental stigma, and instrumental stigma further develops stigma based on symbolic stigma.

While symbolic stigma can be eliminated through conceptual destigmatisation, instrumental stigma is difficult to eliminate once formed. Although it can be gradually weakened, instrumental stigma can easily become entrenched and difficult to eliminate due to the involvement of the interests of people creating the stigma. Thus, it is more difficult to prevent the formation of instrumental stigma and to eliminate it.

5.3 New Changes in Stigmatisation of People Living with HIV/AIDS

With the increasing popularisation of HIV knowledge and extensive publicity against the stigma and discrimination of PLWHA, stigmatisation with a long history in China has undergone new changes. An understanding of the new changes in the stigma against them is conducive to understanding the development and characteristics of HIV stigma and new challenges faced in the new era.

5.3.1 New Changes in People Living with HIV/AIDS

The attitudes of the general public towards AIDS and the mindset of those infected have changed. The sentiment of fear when talking about AIDS has changed considerably.

Firstly, there has been a change in self-identification. PLWHA do not dare to admit openly that they are "sick", but now, some are bold enough to admit it. For instance, if a patient took a taxi to Green Harbour (a ward built by Linfen Infectious Diseases Hospital in 2004), he would only tell the driver that he was going to one village, but now, some patient would tell the driver before getting on the bus, "I am HIV infected and I am going to Green Harbour, do you dare to take on me?" Some kind-hearted drivers would say, "I'll give you a free ride."

Secondly, the pursuit of marriage has changed. In the past, they did not dare to hope for marriage, let alone give birth to children, based on their current status of infection; but now, some not only pursue marriage (getting married with infected people or healthy people), and even expect to have children.

Thirdly, the quest for life has changed. In the past, many suffered a lot psychologically once they learned of their infection and needed to seek professional advice from psychologists. Some may even go to extremes, such as committing suicide. However, now, many have a strong desire to live and are particularly concerned about when they will be cured. For instance, in Shanxi Province, where the idea that "fallen leaves return to their roots" (meaning a person residing elsewhere finally returns to his or her ancestral home) is traditionally valued, when the patients are about to die, their family would like to take them home. Here there are two scenarios: if they are unconscious, nothing will happen; if they are awake, they will be very reluctant to go back, thinking that going back would mean giving up treatment and imminent death.

Fourthly, there has been an improvement in the stability of marriages and a more active pursuit of happiness. In the past, once one person in the family was found to have AIDS, there was a higher probability of choosing to divorce for the other, but now, this has changed considerably.

5.3.2 Widespread Stigma Against People Living with HIV/AIDS

With the widespread publicity of knowledge about AIDS by the state and government, the direct contact of national leaders and public figures with PLWHA, and promising results in medical research on HIV control, society has a clearer understanding of the characteristics, scope and infectivity of the AIDS spread, and discrimination and stigma against AIDS are moving in a favourable direction. However, stigma against PLWHA is still widespread in various forms, although AIDS is no longer seen as a 'super cancer', and the talk of it no longer strikes fear. Despite a significant reduction in outward rejection and a gradual increase in acceptance due to extensive public service campaigns, some studies suggest that the public continues to have an emotional response characterised by strong and unconscious conflicts (Graham et al. 1993).

In general, society still witnesses the prevalent stigma against them and, in particular, more insidious forms of internalised stigma and discrimination with greater difficulty in elimination.

5.3.3 A Shift from Predominantly Symbolic to Instrumental Stigmas

With the deepened understanding of the causes of HIV, there has been a shift from predominantly symbolic stigma to predominantly instrumental stigma in the form of HIV stigma. In the early stages of the AIDS epidemic, the stigmatisation of HIV in China was mainly a literal and direct stigmatisation of the concept of AIDS by authorities, a symbolic stigmatisation that could be transformed to achieve the immediate goal of destigmatisation. In recent years, the value-neutral term "aizibing" (艾滋病) has become the only way of to refer to AIDS in China, which has destigmatised the symbolic stigma against PLWHA. Instrumental stigma, on the other hand, arises from the public's fear of AIDS and is manifested in discrimination against them and their families. The fear of AIDS is still present in society, and instrumental stigma is difficult to eradicate and will persist once formed.

5.3.4 Mutual Stigmatisation of People Living with HIV/AIDS and High-Risk Population

HIV stigma has always been closely linked to high-risk groups for HIV infection, such as prostitutes, homosexuals and drug abusers, who suffer from the same stigma as the HIV community. On the one hand, prior to HIV infection, these groups are themselves subject to social stigma and discrimination. After HIV infection, they have the stigma exacerbated by AIDS and are labelled high-risk groups for HIV infection. On the other hand, the close association of AIDS with these stigmatised groups increases the possibility for stigmatisation of PLWHA.

5.3.5 More Insidious Forms of Stigma: A Shift from the Public to Individuals

HIV stigma has changed from an organisational to an individual act. In the early periods of AIDS in China, the public media reported extensively on the routes of transmission and severity of the disease. The initial stigmatisation began at the public level, where the general public had a stereotype of AIDS through the publicity of authoritative media, a stereotype heavily marked by stigma. Although public media coverage of AIDS has begun to shift from stigmatisation to destigmatisation and from "swatting capitalist flies" to providing care, assistance and support for PLWHA, HIV stigma at the individual level has not been completely eliminated by the authoritative media's caring publicity on AIDS, and the stigma therein is still deeply rooted in many cases. Moreover, individual awareness has not been aligned with authoritative media. Discrimination by organisational behaviour no longer exists, but individual discrimination remains.

5.4 Summary

This chapter adopts literature review and the interview method to sort out and analyse the evolving characteristics and new changes in the stigmatisation of PLWHA, with the aim of gaining a more comprehensive and profound grasp of the forms and changes in the stigmatisation and forming a comprehensive understanding of the stigma therein. Based on social cognitive theory, it analyses symbolic stigma and instrumental stigma and provides different perspectives on the evolution of HIV stigma from the viewpoints of individuals and the general public.

This chapter describes the ways and characteristics of the evolution of symbolic stigma from the perspectives of concept-based symbolic stigma and stigma of vulnerable groups. The conceptual name of AIDS in China has evolved from politically stigmatised "aizibing" (爱资病), to sexually stigmatised "aizibing" (爱滋病), which condemns sexual misconduct, and to value-neutral destigmatised "aizibing" (艾滋病). A conceptual or symbolic destigmatisation of AIDS and PLWHA has been basically achieved in China.

The instrumental stigma (characterised by symptoms of PLWHA), which refers to the fear resulting from lack of adequate information about the symptoms and transmission modes of AIDS, has evolved from scary physical symptoms to manageable physical manifestations in HIV prevention strategies, from incurability to manageability in medical treatments, from physical contacts to fixed modes of transmission in transmission modes, from "sexual-only" transmission to multiple modes of infection in infection modes, and from "blame-oneself-only theory" to "innocence theory" in the basic argument. The symbolic stigma and instrumental stigma form an interactive evolutionary process, with the former providing the basis or tone for the latter and the latter further developing the stigma based on the former.

Finally, after illustrating the new changes in the stigmatisation of PLWHA, this chapter concludes that the stigma therein is still prevalent in society; there is a shift from the predominantly symbolic stigma to the predominantly instrumental stigma; mutual stigma exists between PLWHA and high-risk population; and the more insidious forms of stigma spread from the public to individuals.

References

Graham S, Weiner B, Giulano T, Williams E (1993) An attributional analysis of reactions to magic Johnson. J Appl Soc Psychol 23(9):996–1010
Herek GM (1999) AIDS and stigma. Am Behav Sci 42:1106–1116
Pan S, Huang Y, Li M (2006) The "problems" of AIDS in China explained. Social Sci China 1:85–95

Yao X (2011) The reign of stigma: research on stigma from the perspective of pan-politics, and take AIDS as example. Renmin University of China

Yao X, Wang W (2014) Stigmatisation of AIDS in China in the theoretical perspective of political empathy. J Yunnan Normal Univ (humanities and Social Sciences Edition) 46(4):121–126

Zhou YR (2007) "If you get AIDS, you have to endure it alone": understanding the social constructions of HIV/AIDS in China. Soc Sci Med 65:284–295

Chapter 6
Impact of Stigmatisation and the Destigmatisation of People Living with HIV/AIDS

Stigmatisation is a dynamic process of group interaction in which powerful stigmatisers amplify certain negative characteristics of stigmatised people through labelling until a fixed, unchangeable stereotype is formed (Zhang 2008). HIV stigma stems from the external process of stigmatisation by stigmatisers and the internalisation of stigma by stigmatised people. How HIV stigma manifests itself, how it affects individuals and families, and how it can be destigmatised will be discussed in this chapter.

6.1 Impact of Stigmatisation of People Living with HIV/AIDS

Stigmatisation not only adversely affects PLWHA but also stigmatises their families, destroys their family relationships and even causes harm at a societal level.

6.1.1 Impact on the Individual

6.1.1.1 Serious Psychological Problems

PLWHA have been suffering from HIV physically for a long time and from the threat and stigma of AIDS mentally. Subjected to serious social discrimination, they have problems with their psychological state and behaviours. They suffer from long-term depression, and some even have suicidal tendencies. They generally have more serious psychological problems but have nowhere to pour out or relieve them. Their main manifestations are widespread negative emotions such as fear of AIDS, great psychological stress, depression and pessimism, and even the mentality of revenge against society.

X. Wang, *Destigmatisation of People Living with HIV/AIDS in China*, A Sociological View of AIDS, https://doi.org/10.1007/978-981-16-8534-7_6

1. Fear

PLWHA develop a fear of symptoms of AIDS and HIV stigma once found to be infected with HIV due to the incurability of AIDS and the long-standing social stigma against them. With their mental health seriously affected, many of them have long developed a fear of AIDS and are unable to live a normal life.

> I'm so scared, scared of death, even more scared of a horrible death. Sometimes when the fever doesn't go away, I wonder if it's time to die. If I were to die, I would like to die without pain. The medications don't cure. Anyway, you're just waiting to die if you have AIDS. Medications can only relieve the symptoms. (Infected Case No. 38)

> The doctors say that there is no cure, so it's like giving me a death sentence. I don't know which day I will die. It feels like AIDS will strike any time. (Infected Case No. 39)

> I had heard about but never known about this disease before. I never thought I would get it. I couldn't believe it. It took me a long time to accept it. When I asked others about it, they said there was no cure, and the doctors said there was no cure either. It was then that I started to get scared, knowing that I wouldn't live long and feeling like I was waiting to die. I was so scared that I was in panic every day and refused to meet others. (Infected Case No. 20)

2. Depression

Due to the incurability of AIDS, PLWHA need to take medications for long to control its development. On the one hand, serious social stigma causes them to suffer from physical and mental torture. On the other hand, social stigma causes disruptions in their social relationships, making it difficult for them to receive material and emotional support from their social networks. Consequently, the financial pressure of living, physical suffering and mental stigma and discrimination make them vulnerable to depression.

> I told him not to think too much about it. We would die from any disease sooner or later, right? However, sometimes he just takes things too hard, always thinking AIDS would bring shame on him. Now he doesn't want to go out, or meet others, including his relatives and friends. When I come back from work he would either lie in bed or just sit there, staring blankly. (Non-infected Case No. 20)

> In fact, in the early stages of the disease, I don't have many obvious symptoms. However, I just can't bear the torture in my heart, knowing that there would be no hope of living if I should die sooner or later. What's the point of living if you do not have something to look forward to? (Infected Case No. 39)

> I used to be quite optimistic and cheerful. I loved to joke around, thinking nothing was a problem. Everyone said I was happy every day. However, when I get AIDS, everything is different for me. I feel that I take things too hard. I'm on medication every day. I don't talk about my work or family. I haven't smiled for long. Others may not even know me when seeing me again. (Infected Case No. 27)

3. Suicidal Tendencies

While suffering from AIDS, PLWHA do not gain sympathy and support from others and are discriminated against. Stigma exacerbates their depressive symptoms, and a lack of appropriate outlets for boredom or depression makes them vulnerable to suicidal tendencies.

> When first diagnosed positive, I couldn't eat or sleep. When I lay down I had a messy picture in my mind, which was particularly ugly. The more I thought about it, the more scared I was. I wanted to kill myself and be done with it, but I couldn't leave my son alone. Just let it go. I don't want to think about it anymore. It's useless. I don't care what others say or think about me. (Infected Case No. 32)

> I am a skillful electrician in a factory. I planned to achieve something at work, but I am losing my job and I can't do anything anymore. My home is not like it used to be, and so am I. So why live? I just want to find a place someday where no one knows and take some medicine.... That's it. (Infected Case No. 32)

> I've decided that I'm going to kill myself when it's too late to take the medication in the late stages. I'm sure I can't stand the pain, and it's hard for my family to see it. So I'll just wait and kill myself one day. I don't want to die a horrible death. I've got my cerements ready. I'm not so scared when I think about it. (Infected Case No. 35)

4. Revenging Mentality

In the context of prolonged stigma and discrimination, a small number of PLWHA may develop an extreme mentality of revenge due to the failure to bear the stigma, as in the case of the needle sticking incident in Tianjin Municipality of China in 2002. The revenging mentality they have is a risk factor for social stability and can affect themselves and their families.

> No one greeted me at the banquet in the village. Walking through the village, I saw people with their heads down, pretending not to see me. I sometimes cursed, cursing very badly, saying that if I didn't like anyone, I'd stick needles in them... (Q: Have you truly stuck needles in them?) No, that's not true. I was just angry and upset. (Infected Case No. 17)

PLWHA cannot gain sympathy or care in society but usually feel isolated and rejected due to the increased psychological pressure caused by stigma. Such a social environment creates more psychological problems for them.

6.1.1.2 Concealing the Disease

When PLWHA learn of their infection with HIV, it is initially followed by a great deal of psychological fear and pessimism. Especially in a stigmatised society, they often choose to hide it to protect themselves and their families. They are afraid of being labelled immoral or losing existing social relationships. Most of them are reluctant to disclose their condition to the public, even to their relatives and friends, and some even try to hide it from their spouses and children. It is usually when they have an attack of the disease or have to go to the hospital to take medications for HIV control or when a worker goes to their house for HIV prevention and control that their condition is made public. This accounts for the presence of nearly 800,000 cases in China that are not known (Xiang et al. 2009a).

1. Concealing the Disease From Family Members

PLWHA conceal their illness from their families mainly out of protection for their family members, namely, to relieve the psychological burden on them and to protect their social relationships from being damaged. If the disease is disclosed to family members, family tensions may arise, but prolonged concealment may delay treatment and accelerate the progression of the disease. In addition, family members and relatives or friends do not take precautions to prevent HIV without knowledge of the situation, making them vulnerable to infection within the family.

> My son is quite sensible. At first I hid it from him and said I had the liver disease which was infectious. Later, when he was older and more sensible, I couldn't hide it anymore, so I told him. My son, who always looked worried, didn't say anything when he had something on his mind. However, I could feel that he was in a mood and his academic performance dropped.... (Infected Case No. 35)

> I haven't let my parents know it yet. They're too old to handle it if I tell them. They don't live with us. They live in the countryside with my elder brother, so they can't see me from a distance. I can't let them worry about me at their old age. (Infected Case No. 38)

2. Concealing the Disease From Doctors

Due to medical discrimination in some hospitals, some PLWHA may conceal their illness from doctors for fear of being denied medical treatment or being discriminated against, which makes it easier for doctors to misdiagnose their illness and puts doctors and other patients at risk of infection.

> When I get sick I go to some faraway hospitals. I don't want the doctors and nurses there to know I have AIDS, because some of them without good medical ethics may refuse to treat me. If it's just a minor illness only requiring some medications, I wouldn't say I have AIDS. If it was serious and I had to be put on a drip, I would remind the nurse that I had infectious hepatitis and asked her for attention. The nurse quite gratefully said I was ethical, as some patients wouldn't say anything about their illness. (Infected Case No. 29)

> I don't usually go to the hospital. I just buy some medicines myself if I'm sick. With the extremely low body resistance I fall sick every now and then. I go to the hospital only when I truly have to. All the doctors and nurses at the hospital that I usually visit know me. If it's not convenient, I will go to a faraway clinic or a small private clinic. (Q: Will you tell the doctor about your condition?) I don't tell them, usually don't. I just say it's a minor problem. What's the point of saying that? I basically don't tell them because it only causes trouble. (Infected Case No. 20)

> I usually get the medicine in other places. I don't want to go to local hospitals for medicine. If I do, they'll know everything and I won't choose to see a doctor at the local area. It's convenient to get to Beijing from my place. No one cares about you in Beijing, a big city with a lot of people. It's all programmed. You get your medicine and go home. I think it's quite convenient. The local doctors are not so proficient, and I don't want too many people to know about my illness. I don't mention it when I go to the hospital, and the doctors there usually don't ask about it. It's impossible for the doctor to ask if you have AIDS. I won't say anything about it. If I did, the doctors and nurses and patients would be scared off. (Infected Case No. 29)

stigmatising and discriminatory envir
stigma, developing a pessimistic notio
should be "isolated", and giving up th
stigma, develop self-stigma and discri
from society and social relations.

Research on self-perceived stigma
slowly accept the idea that they are ou
weakened sense of self-esteem (Heath
PLWHA still try to reclaim their digni
perceived stigma and social reality and
of them have slowly accepted the no
HIV stigma neglect the internalisation
such as the social environment and th
misconception that it is the discrimina
and discriminated people always play th
or angry stigmatised people will accep
This is exactly the case. They have in
stigmatised and discriminated against.

> I know the disease is infectious, so I won't g
> why they don't come over. After all, the d
> not they will be infected. (Infected Case N

> When there were weddings and funerals in
> me to, but I usually didn't. I just asked my
> you go, people won't eat with you. So it's
> to be too close. I'm not willing to. They k
> Luckily, I can see them from afar and say

6.1.2 Impact on the Family

The family, as the basic component
financial and emotional support and s
most important support resources for
disrupted, but they are the inevitable
stigma on families is mainly manifest
disruption of family relationships.

6.1.2.1 Stigmatisation of Family M

When the disease of PLWHA is made
regarded as vulnerable groups for HIV
are stigmatised.

Their spouses are required to undergo regular HIV testing and are subjected to isolation and discrimination at work and in society from their colleagues and friends. The impact on their offspring can be long-lasting and far-reaching, which includes limiting their opportunities for normal development, damaging their self-esteem and compromising their trust in others. In particular, their children suffer psychological distress in marriage (as to whether to tell their parents about the disease) and feelings of inferiority.

> Knowing I had HIV, I was worried that my wife would be infected too. After the test she was fine. However, since then she didn't live or eat with me. She felt sorry for me and tried to look after me. I do not want to get her involved, but I'm sure we are distant. (Infected Case No. 33)

> My son is quite sensible. At first I hid it from him and said I had the liver disease which was infectious. Later, when he was older and more sensible, I couldn't hide it anymore, so I told him. My son, who always looked worried, didn't say anything when he had something on his mind. However, I could feel that he was in a mood and his academic performance dropped. He doesn't worry about me. In a rebellious stage, sometimes he yells when he is in a hurry. Why does this happen to me?... (Infected Case No. 35)

> The children in the village call me "Little AIDS", allowed by their parents or grandparents who don't let their children play with me. I got into a fight when I was called that too much. I tell my dad that I want to quit school and go out to work, but he says I'm only in the first year of junior high school, too young to drop out. He still wants me to continue my study, at least until senior high school. (Infected Case No. 37)

6.1.2.2 Disruption of Family Relationships

There are two major family relationships, namely, the relationship between husband and wife and the relationship between parents and children. As the core of a family's stability, the former is crucial to the stability and development of a family, the happiness of individuals and the development of their children. It is damaged by AIDS in two ways: first, it is no longer as close as it used to be due to fear of the infectivity of AIDS; second, it is further distanced or even severely damaged.

> We consulted many data, which told us we won't get infected with adequate precautions even if living together. We were still unsure and thought we should try to avoid sharing things. (Infected Case No. 15)

> It's different from what it used to be. I know the hospital is to blame for his illness, but it has hit our family so hard that it seems to have messed up our lives. We are not rich, but everything was fine. Now he loses his job, and our family's expenses increase. He dare not get too close to me and our child. I could feel he is very miserable indeed. (Non-infected Case No. 46)

> I don't get along with my husband. After I'm infected with HIV, he cares about me no more and thinks it serves me right. He doesn't come home all day, and sleeps in the guest room back home. He doesn't eat at home either. (Q: Where is your child?) The child is sent to live with his parents. My husband and I hardly see each other and he doesn't care about me. So we just get by. (Infected Case No. 18)

6.1.3 *Impact on Society*

As legal citizens of a country, PLWHA should enjoy their rights and perform their duties. In a law-based society, individuals should not be treated unfairly because of a certain disease they have, as this would undoubtedly weaken social integration, undermine the stability and unity of society as a whole, and even damage the public image of the government.

6.1.3.1 Undermining Social Justice and Social Integration

Stigma deprives some members of society of the opportunity to survive and thrive, putting them at a disadvantage, and directly undermines their dignity. Stigma and discrimination undermine social justice and deny PLWHA the rights they deserve. Social discrimination deprives them of the opportunity to work and the basic human rights as citizens and undermines social equity and justice. They also tend to feel alienated from society and have distrustful social attitudes, and in severe cases, they may even develop antagonistic and anti-social feelings.

> Why is the world against me? I haven't done anything to hurt anyone, so why does it happen? I don't want anything special, but only a normal life. I don't have many days left. I just want to live a peaceful life for a few days, but this is not possible. (Infected Case No. 27)

> I have nowhere to express my concern. I've been disappointed for long. I couldn't see it without this. Now I realise that this is the reality. (Infected Case No. 28)

6.1.3.2 Undermining Social Stability and Unity

The stigma and rejection inevitably make PLWHA fight against discrimination. A society with widespread stigma and discrimination against them is bound to have negative factors of social unrest. Fear of AIDS can create social panic and increase social unrest. Rumours about AIDS are often deliberately amplified, distorted and even exaggerated. The disseminated misinformation may cause serious negative social impact of varying degrees.

> I often see reports about AIDS, some of which are not true, describing it as a horrible disease. I believed so at first, but with AIDS for a few years I feel it's actually not scary. Those without the disease don't know, so they are scared. I don't think it's a good idea to publicise it in such a way that it makes people afraid. If you don't know about AIDS, you're afraid. (Infected Case No. 33)

> I think these people need to be properly managed; otherwise, they would definitely get into trouble or take revenge on society. They don't have a job or an income but have an incurable disease. They have no hope in life, afraid of nothing. What if they deliberately infect others with AIDS? What a mess it would be! (Non-infected Case No. 45)

6.1.3.3 Damaging the Image of the Government

In the context of global integration, all countries in the world are faced with the important task of combating AIDS. If the prevention and control efforts of AIDS are not effectively made in China, one of the most important countries in AIDS response, it will directly damage the image of the Chinese government in the international arena. A report from a foreign newspaper reproduced in the November 17, 2001 issue of *Reference News*, a newspaper with the largest circulation in China, openly stated that the Health Commission of Henan Province "bears unshirkable responsibility" for the occurrence and prevalence of AIDS in Henan (Xiang et al. 2009b).

The prevention and control efforts of AIDS have a direct influence on the public's trust in the government. The government's inadequate response to AIDS makes HIV stigma seriously damage the image of the state and the government in the eyes of the public.

> I have nowhere to express my concern. I went to the hospital for a blood transfusion and got AIDS. The government should have good control over these hospitals and forbid them to do such unethical things. They just care about making money and do not mind if the blood is clean or not. There are more accidents in the use of untested blood, and the government must strengthen their administration. (Infected Case No. 36)

> It seems that a lot of people have AIDS now. They are too dangerous. The government must have good control over them. (Non-infected Case No. 46)

> They contract HIV, which is actually none of the business of the government. They have no other people to rely on but the government because they can't afford the treatment. If the government took care of them no more, they would have to wait for death. They have no other choices. (Non-infected Case No. 2)

6.2 Response to Stigmatisation of People Living with HIV/AIDS

There is a need for a concerted response by all parties at all levels to stigma against PLWHA in various forms from various sectors of society. They are required to play a role at the individual, family, community and institutional levels to address the stigma.

6.2.1 Individual Level

At the individual level, they should prevent stigma from being internalised by adjusting their mindset and continue to stimulate their potential to actively participate in anti-stigma activities for a positive response to stigma.

6.2.1.1 Adjusting the Mindset to Prevent Stigma from Being Internalised

Many of them are likely to internalise the stigma of HIV before infection. After infection, they unconsciously internalise the stigma and show a self-destructive or pessimistic mentality or behaviour, losing interest in life and hope for the future. Methods such as protest, education and contact can reduce the stigma of mental illness (Li et al. 2008). In the face of such a dangerous psychological status, positive psychological construction should be carried out by guiding them to adjust their mindset and treat AIDS correctly so as to prevent them from internalising the stigma.

6.2.1.2 Unlocking the Potential of People Living with HIV/AIDS

Infected with HIV, they still have the potential to be developed. We need to change our perception of them by regarding them as people with great potential rather than simply as people in need of protection and help. To change their stigmatised and discriminated status, it is necessary to explore their potential and strengths and encourage and support them in their efforts to improve their self-image, eliminate negative mentalities and build positive images.

Research has found that the greater they are involved in social activities, the greater the amount of emotional, informational and instrumental support they receive (Xiang et al. 2009a). Encouraging and helping them to become actively involved in HIV-related social organisations and activities for a wider range of social activities, enhancing their interpersonal interactions and improving their qualities and abilities will enable them to gain more social capital. Their public stereotype can be changed through positive self-action and an upbeat image to reduce the stigma attached to them.

They should constantly adjust their mindset and face reality positively. For them, to escape the stigma, they must be self-reliant, self-supporting and self-respecting. Only in this way can they gain the respect of the whole society.

> I think I can still do something. I can do some housework at home, as long as I don't get too tired. I can't do things like moving bricks on a construction site, but I can do some general work, like working as a cleaner, sweeping the streets every day. I think I can do it. I really would like to do something, because I'm not that old. If I don't, I'll be useless even if I'm not sick. (Infected Case No. 16)

> We shouldn't deny a person because of this disease. Before it was detected, I was fine. I did what I was supposed to do, and I didn't have any major conditions. After it was detected, I can still do what I need to do. When I really can't do it anymore, that's it. (Infected Case No. 29)

Here, I would like to mention one of my relatives who was infected with HIV through blood transfusions. She did not leave her house for the first few years because of the poverty caused by AIDS. However, with two children who would go to school and get married, she had to face the reality again. Since 2010, she has relied on aquiculture and poultry to support her family, with a net income of 65,000 yuan per year. Others in the village slowly accept her and no longer reject her, especially in public. She has gained respect of most people and reduced the stigma against her by using her wisdom and actions.

6.2.1.3 Encouraging People Living with HIV/AIDS to Actively Fight Against Stigma

The attitudes and actions of stigmatised people have a bearing on the effectiveness of anti-social exclusion and destigmatisation. Social exclusion often results from their active rejection. If they are actively involved in anti-stigma activities, the level of social exclusion and stigma will be significantly reduced (Chen 2009). As victims of stigma, they should change their mindset and rely on themselves and the ASOs to eliminate the stigma against them rather than relying on others for help. It is important that they and their families should be actively involved in the fight against discrimination since all of them suffer from stigma. If they actively spread knowledge of AIDS to those around them, this will help to change public misconceptions about HIV, earn them a greater voice, gain public support and combat HIV.

> (Q: Do you join an ASO?) No, we don't have one here, and no one has approached me. (Q: If there is one, are you willing to join it?) I'm sure I will. There are a lot of patients like me in it, right? Can they help us defend our rights? (Q: Some organisations provide some help for defending rights. Would you like to join it to help more people defend their rights?) Of course I'm willing to. I'm alone and my voice is hardly heard, but a group of people in an organisation have their voices heard. I'm willing to help others defend their rights, which is also helpful for me. There must be such organisations in big cities, but unfortunately here are fewer people who lack the sense of legality, so no one has taken the lead in setting up such an organisation. (Q: Are you willing to?) I can't do it. I can just do odd jobs, but I am not able to manage it. I don't know what to do. It's just okay with me for being an ordinary worker. I think it's a really good organisation. In a similar situation, we can help each other. (Infected Case No. 28)

6.2.2 Community Level

The community plays an increasing role in society. Many scholars argue that the community can provide better support for PLWHA. The community plays an irreplaceable role in disseminating knowledge about HIV prevention and treatment, promoting policy adjustments, assessing HIV-related risk behaviours, promoting appropriate behaviour, reducing negative social impacts of HIV, and providing community care to their families. Community-level support can not only solve a series of difficulties and problems faced by them and their families in a timely and effective manner and improve their quality of life but can also further reduce the medical costs of HIV prevention and treatment. HIV can be addressed by organising and mobilising the community so as to alleviate the financial pressure on the government, prevent and control the spread of HIV and eliminate the stigma and discrimination against PLWHA. Specifically, the community plays its role in the following aspects.

6.2.2.1 Creating an AIDS-Friendly Community Environment

The community is the main area in which PLWHA live. Its humane environment and attitude towards them will have a direct influence on how they feel about stigma. Living in a good community environment helps them regain and build confidence in their lives. An inclusive and friendly community environment provides shelter and necessary support for them. Therefore, communities should strive to become environmentally friendly and actively create a relaxed and humane environment for them.

6.2.2.2 Providing Livelihood Assistance for People Living with HIV/AIDS

Caring for vulnerable people in the community is one of its essential functions. The lack of basic livelihood security can increase the stigma against PLWHA. They often need high medical bills to stay alive, and most of them are incapacitated and find it difficult to afford medical treatment on their own. Addressing the issue of survival is the most pressing need for them, who have to face the enormous pressure to survive. The most basic function of the community is to provide livelihood assistance to them, ensure their basic living and meet their medical care needs. Therefore, the community should give full play to its strengths and mobilise a wide range of forces to provide material and financial assistance to them in an effort to improve their quality of life and eliminate their family worries.

6.2.2.3 Encouraging People Living with HIV/AIDS to Actively Participate in Community Activities

PLWHA reject social activities due to the stigma attached to them and are reluctant to participate in community-based activities (e.g., HIV prevention and control activities). Good community participation can effectively reduce and eliminate the social stigma attached to them and motivate them to actively participate in community activities. Active participation in community activities can, on the one hand, increase opportunities for them to be integrated into the community, enabling them to use community resources, obtain community benefits, increase their interpersonal interaction, obtain support and assistance from the community, and achieve a gradual and positive return to society. On the other hand, it can promote community participation in HIV prevention and treatment activities, creating an atmosphere of universal participation and achieving the effect of eliminating discrimination and stigma against them.

> (Q: Are you willing to participate in activities organised by some community?) No, notices of activities or lectures are often posted on the bulletin board in our community, but I never care about. (Q: Why not?) I don't want to, because I am not welcome to go either. (Q: Will you go if the community workers invite you to?) I don't know. It depends on what the activity is. I don't want to if it's not interesting. (Q: If the community workers invite you to an activity about AIDS prevention and control, are you willing to?) I haven't thought about it. Everyone would know I have AIDS if I went. (Q: How about if your personal information is kept confidential?) That's okay. It's a good thing indeed. (Infected Case No. 22)

It can be seen that they are willing to participate in community activities if the community workers keep their information confidential. The community should actively organise relevant activities to further spread knowledge about HIV prevention and treatment and gradually eliminate stigma.

6.2.2.4 Strengthening the Workforce of Community Workers to Improve Community Service Capacity

For community workers who have direct contact with PLWHA, their knowledge about HIV and attitudes towards the latter represent the basic level of community services for the latter. It is important that communities strengthen their institutions to improve the basic quality and HIV-related knowledge of community workers, as the infected people in the community need help in areas such as livelihoods, basic medical care and psychological counseling. A well-trained professional community workforce is essential for improving their survival and eliminating stigma, which indicates the need to train community workers.

Due to the infectiousness of HIV and the long-standing stigma attached to PLWHA, community services require more resources and further improvement in its service capacity and capability from the community. Communities should not only meet their basic needs and help them overcome the difficulties they face in life but also strive to eliminate the stigma and discrimination against them within the community. In addition, communities should continue to improve their service capacity and carry out relevant activities so as to eliminate stigma and provide better services to them.

6.2.2.5 Promoting Publicity and Training on AIDS

The public's fear and rejection of AIDS stems from a lack of knowledge about the disease. Training and lectures on AIDS should be conducted to dispel the fear of AIDS and PLWHA in the community. This can be done by putting up posters on bulletin boards in the community and distributing materials to actively promote healthy lifestyles and provide information on HIV control and medication. Moreover, the community should provide support for PLWHA in employment and schooling and provide them with education and training in vocational skills so that they are equipped with the means to earn a living.

6.2.3 *Institutional Level*

The Chinese government has always attached great importance to HIV destigmatisation and anti-discrimination efforts to protect the rights and interests of PLWHA and eliminate social discrimination against them. *The Circular on Strengthening Medical Services for People Living with HIV/AIDS* issued by the Ministry of Health of China in 2012 required the implementation of the first diagnosis responsibility system. As a response, all the administrative divisions in Chinese mainland identified and disclosed the list of designated hospitals for AIDS in accordance with the requirements to ensure access to medical care for them.

6.2.3.1 Strengthening Anti-AIDS Stigma Efforts

Public understanding and perceptions of AIDS and PLWHA mainly come from media reports. Thus, the media play an irreplaceable role in combating HIV stigma and helping them cope with social discrimination. Specifically, there are two manageable ways to destigmatise HIV, namely, by creating positive public opinions and using the celebrity effect.

1. Creating Positive Public Opinions

We strengthen collaboration across sectors to further reduce the symbolic stigma of AIDS through publicity of the disease and reduce the instrumental stigma of AIDS through widespread dissemination of knowledge of AIDS prevention and treatment. The news media play a strong role in shaping public opinions. HIV stigma is largely due to biased media coverage and unstandardised wording. The public learns about AIDS and forms a basic understanding of AIDS mainly through the media, such as television, newspapers and the internet. Thus, it is important for the news media to direct public opinions correctly towards the destigmatisation of PLWHA. The first thing to do for the media is to present an objective image of them and report accurately and fairly on them so as to guide others to view them correctly.

Since the first case of HIV infection was discovered in China in 1985, there have been increasingly more news reports about HIV, through which the majority of the public has learned about AIDS. They have played a vital role in disseminating knowledge about HIV prevention, shaping the image of PLWHA and creating a social environment conducive to HIV prevention and treatment. Moreover, the media have played a key role in eliminating the stigma and discrimination against PLWHA, and taken the right direction in consciously eliminating negative labels associated with them and removing the veneer of immorality from AIDS. It is the unshirkable responsibility of the media to describe their image as patients in need of special care, treatment and assistance.

Therefore, in the publicity of AIDS, first, the media should be called upon to report on AIDS events in a scientific, rigorous, accurate and objective manner, to widely disseminate knowledge about AIDS prevention, minimise the negative impact of the reports, and enhance the public's awareness of destigmatisation of HIV and sense of social responsibility. Second, medical experts, sociologists and psychologists should be invited to strictly scrutinise publicity and education materials to ensure their scientificness, objectiveness and accuracy, remove or replace stigmatising language and labels, and create a favourable social environment for AIDS prevention and treatment.

2. Using the Celebrity Effect

The celebrity effect should be used in destigmatising PLWHA. The National Health and Family Planning Commission (now the National Health Commission of China) has included celebrities such as Peng Liyuan, Pu Cunxin, Zhou Tao and Jiang Wenli among its AIDS prevention campaigners. They have actively participated in anti-discrimination activities as public figures and guided the public in the proper understanding and treatment of PLWHA by using the celebrity effect. Reports of these celebrities' contact with PLWHA have been publicised to eliminate HIV stigma. In general, this has had a positive effect on AIDS destigmatisation. In addition, through the public screening of public service films about AIDS directed by celebrity directors, relevant authorities have promoted their positive image in fighting HIV and called on all sectors of society to care for and help rather than discriminate against them.

6.2.3.2 Providing Social Support for People Living with HIV/AIDS

The "Four Frees and One Care" policy introduced in China in 2006 is one of the most powerful policy measures in the fight against AIDS. The "Four Frees" policy covers PLWHA in rural areas and those economically disadvantaged people in urban areas not covered by basic medical insurance who receive and take free antiretrovirals at hospitals for infectious diseases designated by the health authorities or at general hospitals with infectious disease departments, people voluntarily coming for HIV counselling and testing who receive free counselling and primary screening at designated hospitals and disease prevention and control centres at all levels, pregnant women infected with HIV who are provided with health counselling, childbirth services and free drugs blocking mother-to-child transmission by local designated hospitals, and orphans of PLWHA who are provided with psychological rehabilitation services and free compulsory education by local governments. The policy is concerned not only with how to provide medical assistance to them but also with how to solve problems in the psychology and education of their children or orphans. It provides comprehensive social support to them physically and mentally, shows humanistic care for them, and plays an important role in preventing the formation of self-stigma and promoting the independent personality of their children or orphans.

The care and support for them mainly depends on social assistance provided by the government at all levels, which shows that the social support policies implemented by the government have favourable social effects. However, the mobile population still has difficulties in accessing AIDS-related welfare support and services. Thus, efforts should be made to provide more support for them in relevant welfare benefits and services and include them within the AIDS welfare service system to provide positive social support, alleviate their plight and mental pressure, and provide policy and financial support to help them address stigma in an ultimate effort to destigmatise stigma.

6.2.3.3 Eliminating Discrimination Against People Living with HIV/AIDS in Access to Health Care and Schooling Through Institutional Means

PLWHA are generally subject to undue discrimination in access to health care and schooling, which involve their most direct interests and fundamental rights. Thus, it is the most pressing need for them to eliminate discrimination in access to health care and schooling.

1. Eliminating Discrimination in Access to Health Care

PLWHA need long-term medication due to the physical destruction caused by AIDS. Thanks to the "Four Frees and One Care" policy introduced in China in 2006, they can receive antiretrovirals for treatment free of charge. Nonetheless, some hospitals show behavioural and attitudinal discrimination in access to health care, such as refusing to provide medical services to them, refusing to hospitalise them, treating them indifferently and avoiding them deliberately, which brings negative effects such as inconvenience in accessing health care and psychological stress to them.

To address discrimination in access to health care, the health authorities should further introduce policies to improve the service standards of hospitals, provide training to hospital staff on professional ethics, and adopt clear rules and regulations to regulate the actions and words of health care workers to eliminate discrimination in access to health care against PLWHA.

2. Eliminating Discrimination in Schooling

The right to education is a fundamental right of children in China. It is unfair to be denied the right to education because of AIDS for children with AIDS and the minor children of PLWHA who are the most vulnerable to discrimination in schooling.

The main reasons for the discrimination against PLWHA in schooling lie in the fear of AIDS on the part of schools, teachers, students and their parents, lack of understanding of the pathology and transmission modes of AIDS, and the prejudice and stereotyping of AIDS. To eliminate discrimination in schooling against children with AIDS and children of PLWHA, schools should be called upon to hold regular lectures on AIDS, put up posters about AIDS, advocate teachers and students to actively learn about AIDS prevention, improve care and support for them, create an inclusive and friendly school atmosphere, and ensure their right to education in an effort to eliminate the HIV stigma at the childhood stage.

6.2.3.4 Expanding the Channels of Expressing the Interests of People Living with HIV/AIDS

It is a common phenomenon in society that PLWHA, as a vulnerable group, lack channels to express their interests and are unable to defend their rights. To free them from stigma, it is crucial that their rights, as clearly defined in the laws and regulations, are granted and realised, so that they can clearly express their legitimate interests (Shen 2005).

1. Repealing Policies Discriminating Against People Living with HIV/AIDS

The issue of legislation on HIV discrimination has been of concern to the academic and legal communities. Although HIV stigmatisation is often considered informal, there is legal and overt discrimination against PLWHA in reality, mainly including restrictions on travel, mandatory isolation, and compulsory testing and reporting, which is in effect a restriction on their fundamental rights and freedoms. Most countries and regions have realised that it is unfair to restrict their rights and freedoms (Malcolm et al. 1998). It is imperative that policies that discriminate against them should be repealed and protective laws and regulations should be enacted, which is of great significance to HIV destigmatisation.

2. Establishing Specialised Rights Advocacy Bodies for People Living with HIV/AIDS

PLWHA, as a vulnerable group, are not granted many rights by the system, and the existing rights they have are difficult to safeguard due to a variety of factors. Thus, special institutions should be established to safeguard their basic rights. There are occasional cases of jeopardised rights and interests in providing assistance to them, such as untimely assistance, discrimination in employment and schooling. In such cases, most of them are not aware of their rights or cannot find channels to defend them. Special departments should be set up in AIDS prevention and treatment institutions to provide a channel for them to express and defend their interests, help them safeguard their legitimate rights and interests, and realise their basic human rights.

3. Supporting AIDS Service Organisations to Fight for Their Voices

As is known to all, the influence of individuals is always limited, and social organisations can fight for their rights on behalf of them. The government should actively encourage PLWHA to set up and join ASOs and make their voices heard in society. The stigma can be hopefully eliminated by safeguarding their basic rights, opposing discrimination and exclusion of them, and expanding the influence of ASOs.

6.3 Summary

Using interview data and qualitative research methods, this chapter focuses on the negative impact of HIV stigma on PLWHA and society and discusses how HIV stigma manifests itself, how it affects individuals and families and how HIV destigmatisation is achieved.

This chapter focuses on the impact of and responses to the stigma of PLWHA and addresses the stigma and discrimination against them in the mental, working, medical care, schooling and other areas. Stigma affects them at the individual, group and social levels. At the individual level, it causes chronic fear, depression and, in many cases, suicidal ideation and revenge among them. It also causes them to conceal their illness from their families and friends, which has more serious consequences. It also leads to the destruction of social networks and loss of social capital, which leads to further internalisation of stigma and self-loathing. At the group level, the impact is shown in the stigmatisation of family members and destruction of family relationships. At the social level, the HIV stigma undermines social justice, stability and unity, weakens social integration, and even damages the image of the government.

How PLWHA should respond to stigma from various sectors of society in various forms at the individual, family, community and institutional levels is an issue that needs to be addressed for long periods of time. At the individual level, they should actively adjust their mindset to prevent stigma from being internalised, stimulate their potential and actively participate in anti-stigma activities. At the community level, it is important to create an AIDS-friendly community environment, conduct AIDS-related publicity and training, and encourage them to actively participate in community activities. At the institutional level, the anti-AIDS stigma campaign should be strengthened by creating positive public opinions and using the celebrity effect to provide social support and broaden the channels for them to express their interests and demands.

Of course, as a sociological researcher, the author is well aware that the policy recommendations or ideas to combat stigma are still largely idealistic and "contingent" arguments. Nevertheless, this is the very historic mission of all researchers (including the author) to strive for HIV destigmatisation.

References

Chen Q (2009) Border and return: the study on social exclusion of PLWHA. Social Sciences Academic Press

Heatherton Told F, Kleck Robert E (2000) The social psychology of stigma. The Guilford Press

Li Q, Gao M, Xu D (2008) Review of theories on the development of mental illness stigma. Adv Psychol Sci 16(4):582–589

Malcolm A, Aggleton P, Bronfman M, Galvao J, Mane P, Verrall J (1998) HIV-related stigmatization and discrimination: its forms and contexts. Crit Publ Health 8(4):347–370

Shen Y (2005) Empowerment at the bottom is most important in building a "harmonious society." Inform Decisions Magazine 1:19

Xiang D et al (2009a) Need and response: social support for PLWHA. Social Sciences Academic Press

Xiang D et al (2009b) Difficult position and way out: social predicament of PLWHA. Social Sciences Academic Press

Zhang Y (2008) Stigmatisation situations and their coping strategies: a case study of urban adaptation and community change among migrants. Society 4:126–147

Chapter 7
Ways to Destigmatise People Living with HIV/AIDS: Practice and Inspirations

AIDS has always been around us but has been ignored because it has no immediate threat. In their studies on AIDS prevention and control, researchers hold that HIV stigma is no longer a purely social issue but may turn into an occurrence of stigma against PLWHA by individuals or groups, deepening the antagonism between groups and worsening the situation of overall social governance. They attempt to correlate the seemingly different academic fields, for instance, to explore whether the formation of such stigma is related to the stereotypes and fears that have existed for a long time, the failure of education, misinformation in the media, moral chains, discrimination and prejudice, bias in law enforcement, lack of laws, and injustice in the administration of justice. Some of these factors contribute to the fear of HIV stigma, the prejudice that HIV is a special disease, or even that PLWHA are punished for breaking taboos and precepts. As a result, the ingrained inexplicable hatred results in hatred, prejudice and discrimination against them by individuals or groups. When building up to a certain level, it becomes an outlet for each other, and they become innocent victims. In particular, when hate incidents occur, the horrific coverage by some of the media often leads to misunderstandings among the general public, reinforcing their discrimination against and fear of PLWHA.

7.1 Challenges/Barriers to Destigmatisation of People Living with HIV/AIDS

7.1.1 Lack of Knowledge About HIV: Primary Barrier to Destigmatisation

Overall, there is a general lack of knowledge of AIDS among the public. During the interviews, the author found that the interviewees mostly had a smattering of AIDS-related knowledge and did not have a good understanding of infection by other means

X. Wang, *Destigmatisation of People Living with HIV/AIDS in China*, A Sociological View of AIDS, https://doi.org/10.1007/978-981-16-8534-7_7

of transmission, such as deep kissing or oral sex, and the perception, presence and treatment of adverse consequences of multiple sexual partners. Only approximately 10% of the public believe that the current information on promoting condoms for HIV prevention is sufficient; the main sources of information are TV commercials, news and computer networks. In the future, the government should strengthen its publicity and guidance on the transmission routes of HIV (clarifying the transmission routes with different partners at different stages), prevention methods (emphasising the effect of condom use on personal hygiene, prevention of pregnancy and diseases such as HIV), morbidity (requiring self-examination of previous sexual experiences and informing ways to contract HIV) and treatment (reducing side effects of taking medication, and impact on quality of life and future career planning). These are the keys to our future efforts in the effective intervention in HIV prevention and control.

Only 20% of people with multiple sex partners always used condoms in the past and are willing to always use condoms in the future. Thus, there is still much room for the government to promote condom use in HIV prevention, for instance, by using the most popular media such as TV commercials, news and computer networks.

It is recommended to further evaluate previous approaches, methods and contents of publicity on HIV and condoms to revise the contents and strategies of future interventions. Previous sources of information on HIV and condoms have not significantly influenced people's attitudes towards HIV, condoms and their behavioural intentions to use condoms during sex and have not achieved the desired effect on HIV prevention.

As behavioural change depends on changes in previous perceptions and attitudes, the aforementioned recommendations of people's in-depth knowledge of HIV and condoms will influence their attitudes towards HIV and condoms and reduce barriers to condom use, which in turn will influence their behavioural intentions for future condom use.

In addition, it is recommended that PLWHA should be chosen as spokespersons for the future publicity of condom use to raise awareness of HIV prevention through their personal experiences to influence future behaviour towards condom use during sex.

The attitudes of those who always used condoms during sex towards condoms will be a very important cue for intervention in future publicity, and the media could be used to raise public awareness of condom use.

The publicity of HIV prevention indicates the need to understand relevant knowledge and make some change in attitudes, which must be done through situational guidance. Thus, the author would like to make some suggestions on the connotation of promoting condom use for HIV prevention.

Firstly, we can include HIV-related knowledge in the publicity and consider using celebrities and cartoon characters as spokespersons to teach people about condom use during sex to stimulate discussion about condom use and encourage people to prepare condoms for their first sex and to use them correctly and throughout.

Secondly, we can design specific scenarios, for instance, where both partners honestly say that they have had partners before or where one partner makes a claim that condom use during sex is a new fashion trend by emphasising the serious consequences of condomless sex. Of course, it is important to that although men and women love and trust each other, they should hold the responsibility for persistent condom use, which is a way to protect and love each other. That is, condoms are considered fashionable because using them is a way of showing responsibility and a sign of love for each other.

Finally, we should emphasise the benefits of condom use by promoting the notion that it increases sexual pleasure and interest to reduce the psychological barriers to it. Moreover, both partners are more comfortable and happier during sex without the threat of disease and pregnancy concerns.

Through the aforementioned advertising and publicity with similar contents and scenarios, the interventions of cognitive, attitudinal and behavioural change can be used as a reference for future promotion of condom use for HIV prevention. It is also recommended that relevant studies should be conducted to evaluate the content, process and outcome of the intervention strategies with a view to contributing to the prevention of AIDS.

7.1.2 Repeated Drug Abuse: Challenge to Destigmatisation

Effectively reducing the number of drug abusers is one of the most important ways to tackle the spread of HIV. The government should ensure that the community-based prevention and treatment functions of drug abuse prevention and control centres are fulfilled in all its departments. In addition, correctional institutions should work with outstanding private drug rehabilitation centres to establish a control system for detoxifying drug abusers in the community and to build a network of "medical-patient relationships" within the community.

In his research, the author found that drug abusers almost always believe they cannot resist the temptation of drug addiction, which shows their compromised confidence in detoxification. Therefore, the government and medical centres should actively provide assistance and support for drug rehabilitation when drug abusers need the care of others most instead of stopping providing all resources when their addiction is disclosed. This is because the moment a drug abuser takes drugs again is the beginning of the peak of hidden problems; if the demon of drug addiction cannot be overcome at this time, the entire support for drug rehabilitation will end in failure.

The increase in the number of drug abusers is bound to have a negative impact on the fight against AIDS. Establishing drug rehabilitation control of drug abusers in the community and linking them to the medical network upon their return to society is a crucial task. As shown in the author's research, most drug abusers feel that psychological counselling helps them kick the addiction and that they have high expectations for drug rehabilitation and are eager to receive professional psychological counselling during the support period. In addition, they are very interested in and have a high demand for HIV prevention and treatment courses delivered in the community. These two needs is simply a desire for help. The lack of willpower is a personality trait of them, who often have an avoidant attitude faced with major changes in their lives. Thus, it would be most helpful if they should be provided with the psychological counselling and medical resources they need when returning to society.

A high proportion of drug abusers do not have confidence in drug rehabilitation or would like drug rehabilitation centres to provide courses and resources related to drug rehabilitation and HIV prevention and control to help them kick the habit. Nevertheless, there has been a lack of private centres for drug rehabilitation in China, whether in terms of the adequacy of medical facilities, professionalism of drug rehabilitation practitioners, legitimacy of medical procedures for drug rehabilitation, applicability of the constructed drug rehabilitation models, openness of community-based drug rehabilitation resources, or the identification of effectiveness of drug rehabilitation. The work of drug rehabilitation is daunting, and the cooperation between a few hospitals and correctional institutions alone is absolutely not enough. Relevant regulatory bodies should expeditiously legalise the incentives for drug rehabilitation practices and actively encourage private hospitals with drug rehabilitation expertise to join the ranks of drug rehabilitation to expand China's drug rehabilitation services and enable drug abusers to quit drugs in drug rehabilitation centres of a certain scale.

Currently, some people are on the edge of the law by privately providing "detoxification drugs" to drug abusers in the name of detoxification. Nevertheless, there is a lack of strong and timely monitoring by the government's medical management departments, resulting in varying qualities of private drug detoxification centres. Drug abuse prevention and control centres have been set up across China to take on management roles, but the progress of drug rehabilitation operations is hampered by funding difficulties, a lack of staff on the regular payroll and too many part-time staff. In the case of tracking and counselling operations for drug addicts, private drug detoxification centres can hardly provide resources to relevant agencies and have not achieved significant results in drug detoxification. Thus, it is essential and pragmatic to find ways to encourage private professional medical institutions or teaching institutions to assist drug abusers in reintegrating into society.

The insignificant results of drug detoxification make the chances of preventing the spread of AIDS unlikely. Prevention of AIDS and control of drug abuse must go hand in hand to effectively contain the spread of AIDS. The medical issues that PLWHA need to face in the process of institutional support include the establishment of medical relationships, the presence of medical resources in the community, medical approaches and medical ethics. However, the author's research is still lacking in healthcare administration theories and medical resources, and further research by other experts with medical backgrounds is needed.

7.2 Resources and Platforms Available for Destigmatisation of People Living with HIV/AIDS

7.2.1 Support for Destigmatising Families of People Living with HIV/AIDS is Equally Important

After the confirmed diagnosis of AIDS among PLWHA, their families also face the discrimination and trauma because HIV stigma not only hurts themselves but is deeply embedded in the minds of their families. There is no difference in such stigma between Western and Chinese cultures, as it has social and cultural connotations.

HIV can be transmitted through sex and is first discovered in homosexuals. Thus, they are seen as a high-risk group for AIDS, given a negative and deviant cultural meaning and even considered to be "condemned" for having AIDS. In other words, AIDS is seen not only as a disease but also as a sin.

This study found that shame attached to stigma was present in the life experience of parents of each person living with HIV/AIDS. Their parents felt stigmatised in a wide range of ways, from rejection by family members, alienation by friends, rejection by medical personnel, to non-acceptance by society at large. In general, the information about AIDS and the stigma attached to it come largely from the mass media, especially the news media. It was clear from the interviews that their parents' knowledge and impressions of AIDS also came from media reports.

The news media is a double-edged sword. On the one hand, the coverage of AIDS provides a general description of knowledge about HIV prevention and treatment; on the other hand, the way it presents the news can be an enhancer of stigma. For instance, early media coverage of AIDS-related issues was inevitably mixed with panic and confusion; there were biased reports on how HIV was transmitted among sex workers and homosexuals; and there were focused reports on the rejection and stigmatisation of PLWHA in certain communities. All these have reinforced the perceived horror of the disease and increased social stigma and discrimination. As a result, their parents believe that this is where stigma and discrimination come from.

7.2.2 The Media's Construction of Images of People Living with HIV/AIDS Concerns the Effectiveness of Destigmatisation

One of the prerequisites for exploring issues related to PLWHA is the need to identify the link between the mass media and other social structures, and a systemic perspective helps clarify their relationship. Scholars in China hold that information about PLWHA is not directly produced by the mass media but is first absorbed and then processed in a particular systemic way by the mass media guided by "curiosity". The process cannot be explained or supported from a medical viewpoint, nor can it be explained within the system of the doctor-patient relationship. However, it becomes a "known" thing and a "demand for further information" through a mechanism constructed within the system and becomes a continuous process of communication in public discussion. This in turn affects the environmental systems, such as the policy-making system and the medical system, thus facilitating the link between the mass media and other social structures. It is important to note, however, that this is only a link between the mass media system and other social structures; the mass media itself cannot construct a consensual knowledge system, as the diversity of information increases with social differentiation, further affecting the stability of its systemic reconstruction.

It can be understood through a systemic perspective that there is a conflict between social and media systems for the construction of media, which is hidden behind the media message. The media system produces its self-involving message within the conflict between the various social systems, and this message in turn influences the social system and further influences the extent of its discrimination.

Most notably, curiosity about homosexuality has contributed to the focus of attention on HIV and PLWHA in the news media. In early cases, AIDS was mostly seen as a disease carried by foreigners, and Chinese people were presented as a group in need of protection. In the late 1990s when the AIDS epidemic in some of China's coastal cities became more severe, drug abusers and homosexuals became the main others. A number of journals have tended to believe that homosexuals are HIV carriers and that nonhomosexuals become the ones in need of protection. When heterosexuals outnumber homosexuals in HIV infection, the argument that homosexuals are scapegoats is no longer held true in popular culture, allowing women seen as promiscuous in the dominant culture (mainly sex workers) to be reconfirmed as the others.

In the mass media, there is a bias that distance from others could be constructed and consolidated either through prompt institutionalisation or moral criticism. As a result, due to the ignorance of opinions of citizen groups, the majority of people always regard PLWHA as the source and cause for others' infection with HIV and have an avoidant attitude towards them. The others constructed include foreigners, gay men, bisexuals, sex workers, sexually diverse women, and those at risk of mother-to-child transmission, among others. Such construction can be seen as the main process of marginalisation, where power operates to define the cultural attributes of others to achieve social control.

7.2.3 The Internet Provides an Important Platform for AIDS-Related Organisations in Efforts for Destigmatisation

This study focuses on the impact of the internet on the available capital of non-governmental organisations (NGOs) and on citizens' access to knowledge. In order to gain a deeper understanding of these two impacts of the internet, the author chose to examine single cases and multi-platform examples of social organisation support.

The author found that the websites of AIDS-related organisations largely focused on care for others and were significantly less able to mobilise online and use the structural capital available within the community than other organisations within the network. After examination of the attributes of these organisations, the study found that the organisations at the centre of the network were supported by strong economic and social resources. In contrast, some organisations such as the AIDS Association sponsored by some NGOs still lack the support of social forces. This may be inferred as a lack of social capital, contributing to the gap in cyberspace resources.

Even among the highly marginalised group of PLWHA, there is still "secondary marginalisation" within the group. It is clear from the interviews that they are able to maintain their lives in the same way as others as long as they take medications and have check-ups regularly. Nevertheless, some NGOs are AIDS transit agencies, which can be readily identifiable. In such cases, PLWHA avoid direct contact with them to avoid being identified and even adopt a self-protective approach such as anonymity online. It seems clear that there is a gap in network resources between those who are "infected but healthy" and those who are "infected and need support"; the latter and the organisations that serve them seem to be marginalised once again.

The study also found that AIDS-related organisations and homosexual-related organisations as the channel for information dissemination and mobilisation often established legitimacy by bringing together more people with common experiences of vulnerability. In this way, the issue is raised from the level of rights of individuals to that of rights of the disadvantaged group. In light of this, it is possible to identify the mobilisation strategy of AIDS-related organisations in tandem with homosexual-related organisations. Although the organisations are in tandem with each other, they avoid the words "drug abuse" and "homosexuality" in their discourse and emphasise the use of more neutral or less socially taboo terms such as "facts of AIDS" to gain more support. In other words, PLWHA are still unable to avoid the marginalising tendency of the mainstream media even in cyberspace and have to avoid any negative perceptions in their wording strategies.

Given that the mobilisation strategy favours the disadvantaged group, how does it affect the general public? It is clear from the interview data that online texts can simply provide a richer range of information. While it is true that the disadvantaged groups are more responsive on the internet, the public is more engaged in offline activities. It can be seen that the gay community and socially active PLWHA still avoid the risk of being identified, confine their supporting activities to the internet but do not participate in offline activities. As a result, the internet has not been able to fully resist the marginalisation strategies of the mainstream media and history of stigmatisation. Social mobilisation must still rely on organisations with shared experience of others, and the network is unable to fully change the perception of mainstream values in terms of wording strategies.

Moreover, real social capital affects online technological capital, and the NGOs in the interview have to rely on organisations with government backgrounds as a platform for the integration of online resources. This feature is arguably the strength of the internet. While the lack of real social capital cannot be changed, subjects can be kept from being silenced through online connections, and counselling can be disseminated through other websites.

The function of information dissemination of the internet also has age differences. For respondents over 30 years of age, the main source of information is the mainstream media, and the internet is mainly used as a way to search for further information. For respondents over 20 years of age, however, the internet acts as a warning and offers different forms of support, including film production and music composition.

However, the anonymity of the internet still does not remove the fear of being identified among users. This may be because the NGOs have taken too strong a stance and that PLWHA and homosexuals have avoided direct contact with them to avoid being identified. Even when contact is needed, they apply for a separate account, which is inconsistent with people's optimistic expectations of the internet. Even under the great influence of the internet, the most important factors influencing the trend of the issue and the willingness to participate are the taboo nature of the issue and the possibility of being identified.

7.3 Disclosure of the Identity of People Living with HIV/AIDS

In August 2016, the media reported that 15 of the 16 candidates with AIDS from the Linfen Red Ribbon School in Shanxi Province had been admitted to university. There are two views on the internet on whether their identity should be made public or not. One view holds that it should not be disclosed because these children have been under great pressure since birth and have managed to get into university through their own efforts. If their identities are disclosed, they will inevitably be viewed differently by their classmates, teachers and society as a whole, which will certainly have a great impact on their psychology and physiology. Those who hold the opposite view point out that if their identities are concealed, there is a risk of infecting others in the university because those healthy people also have the right to know about the hidden insecurities that may exist around them.

The word "AIDS" was first associated with sexual misconduct, and the relatively quick death associated with HIV infection fuelled fears among the public. Today, we know about the ways in which HIV is transmitted (blood, sex, mother-to-child transmission) in the publicity of the health authorities, nonprofit organisations and other media and seem to believe we can avoid it if we are not involved in these three ways. Relevant medical and research institutions also constantly release information that AIDS is a chronic disease whose viral load is well controlled, and the life expectancy of infected people is much longer.

Despite this, we cannot effectively address the issue of AIDS.

7.3.1 Widespread Stigma in the Society We Live in

Within the same community, people often have the same perceptions and patterns of thinking, feeling, speaking and acting because they share the same patterns of language use and value systems and ideologies. If you are a man, you should be strong; a slender man with a curvy body may be rejected by others, for instance, be labelled insulting terms such as "unmanly". If you are poor, perhaps this is because you come from a poor background or because of a natural or man-made disaster, but in the eyes of other social groups, poverty results from laziness. The value reflected in discussions such as the one entitled "Should subsidies and benefits for the poor be removed to motivate them to advance" is constructed in language use patterns. You are rich, maybe because you are hard-working or have seized a good opportunity, but those from relatively poorer social groups always believe the wealth of the rich is ill-gotten and earned by trampling on rules and morals. People often believe their familiar patterns of language use refer to something as an objective fact and forget that the so-called "fact" is the product of constructing discursive processes.

When faced with stigma, most of these groups are able to recover after a short period of anger. The general public also finds the process of stigmatisation uninteresting and ends it abruptly. Why did the admission of 15 HIV-infected students to the university cause such extreme panic among some people?

7.3.2 Social Context of Stigmatisation of AIDS and People Living with HIV/AIDS

7.3.2.1 Medical Analysis

Unlike other marginalised groups, PLWHA construct and acquire their identity based on their physical "pathological heterogeneity". This physical transformation is the root cause of the transformation of their identity. Their identity initially comes from the diagnosis and professional knowledge of AIDS, a relatively new infectious disease.

Most of the early diagnoses of PLWHA in China came from medical screening. Although the disease was already present and had serious consequences, this pure pathological phenomenon was not associated with their identity due to a lack of common sense. It was not until HIV infection was discovered in batches during a screening that the disease first became known to the public. The infectious, incurable and lethal characteristics of HIV were known as part of medical and health care knowledge, which became the initial source of information and the decisive basis for constructing their identity. Thus, they were first defined as people who carried the lethal virus.

As a new type of disease, AIDS is incurable worldwide, whose specificity makes medical interventions a necessity in their daily lives and implicitly contributes to the construction of their identity. For them, receiving treatment means that taking medications becomes a daily habit, and their identity changes from "normal people" to "patients". This identity as patients is clearly long-term and irreversible and brings about the "pathological transformation" in social identity.

At the same time, constructed by the patterns of medical language use, they are long-term and debilitated "patients" as well as dangerous "infectious patients". This construct is ironically present in their treatment, and the stigmatised identity is reinforced by the "professionalism" of the constructors.

Initially, the construction of the identity of PLWHA was medical in nature, and the construction of medical knowledge became the reference and foundation for other socially constructive forces. The power of "professionalism" was so strong that practitioners amplified the negative features of HIV and made behavioural choices that did not meet professional requirements. Because of the importance of professional power in the construction of knowledge and the pattern of power, this construction is perceived as a pointer to the fact that patients who doctors are unwilling to deal with become an inherent image of PLWHA, and their stigmatised status is clearly reinforced by medical forces.

In summary, the medical forces rely on their body of knowledge and the resulting patterns of language use to construct a series of identities such as "infected with HIV", "infectious", "vulnerable" and "dangerous". Thus, the identity as "stigmatised" of PLWHA is visible.

In 2016, approximately 38 million cumulative cases of HIV infection survived worldwide, among which half of the cases were treated with antiretroviral therapy and achieved efficacy, effectively curbing the AIDS epidemic. Prioritised treatment was proposed as a means of preventing and controlling AIDS at the 20th International AIDS Conference held in Melbourne, Australia in July 2014. The expansion of HIV treatment was formally proposed to be used as a prevention strategy, calling on governments to act together at the 21st International AIDS Conference held in Durban, South Africa in July 2016. In 2016, the WHO developed the 90-90-90 strategy for accelerated implementation of AIDS prevention and control from 2016 to 2021 and planned to end the epidemics of AIDS, viral hepatitis and other infectious diseases by 2030 based on the advice of The Joint United Nations Programme on HIV/AIDS (UNAIDS) and relevant departments (WHO 2016). These plans and strategies have been proposed to make AIDS a treatable and manageable infectious disease from a medical perspective.

7.3.2.2 Others' Speculation and Image Demonisation: Cultural Trials and Stigma

Here, we can use the subject construction perspective proposed by Pan Suiming and Huang Yingying to explore the phenomenon. In their view, the stigmatiser is the active subject, and the phenomenon (stigmatisation and exclusion of PLWHA) is the result of the subject's construction (rather than something that exists naturally or is only environmentally determined). This perspective focuses more on the construction processes (rather than the results and effects of the construction) based on the subject's feelings and experiences (rather than the researcher's perceptions). The material chosen by the author comes from comments on the website of Zhihu (a Chinese platform similar to Quora) on whether or not the identity of AIDS students should be disclosed. Let us look at how several commenters on the Zhihu website have constructed this phenomenon, which can be roughly summarised as follows.

Firstly, the following commenters believe AIDS is "absolutely incurable":

> AIDS is so terrifying because of its 'absolutely incurable' nature. Once you're infected, there's no escape. Every person infected or every carrier of the virus is a bomb. It would be unfair to others to hide this information.
>
> People with AIDS are as much a beast as AIDS. Like leprosy, AIDS is incurable. We would still be terrified of it even if we knew 100% about it. Thanks to the country's great publicity, people don't deliberately discriminate against PLWHA, but they still avoid them because of fear.

Secondly, they believe the stigma is based on the concern that it is possible that others will get HIV when staying with students with HIV due to "uncontrollable" factors. Look at the following comments.

> Humans are naturally selfish. If these people who fall in love with others do not tell them this information before the relationship is started but rather tell them after it has stabilised or simply keep it to themselves, their lovers are not guilty. Right? Even if all of them are of good character and do not intentionally harm others, who will be to blame if others who don't know this get injured and cross-infected in an accident?
>
> Ordinary students will inevitably be exposed to students with AIDS. Although this is generally not contagious, there is no guarantee that no HIV in their body fluids or blood will invade others' bodies. How should it be handled if an AIDS-infected student is injured and bleeding? It will probably cause chaos in the dormitory.
>
> Should a student infected with AIDS speak out his mind to his lover if he has one? However, there should be no intimate contact because even broken oral mucosa can be extremely dangerous.
>
> There is inevitable contact if they live together. Even if they have a clear mind, others may be infected if they do not know. Although such probability is small, it does not mean that it will never happen. If such a thing happens, who is to blame? Who should see justice done for the victims?
>
> HIV can be transmitted through direct contact with mucosa in the mouth, genitals, anus, etc. or blood, semen, vaginal secretions, or breast milk infected with the virus. This means that it is a very high risk to live with a student infected with HIV. It is common for guys at universities to share a bottle of water or to use a friend's cup. If the friend happens to be a carrier of HIV and you happen to have a mouth ulcer, you have a very high chance of infection. If a person with the virus meets a girl he loves, will he give up his pursuit? Or will he make that girl infected with HIV so that she has no other choice?

Thirdly, they argue that while the 15 HIV-infected students have the right to education, the right to information should also be a fundamental right of non-infected students; the first way to avoid contracting HIV is to be informed about it. Thus, disclosure of identity is not a stigma. For example, here are some comments: "If I were one of their classmates, I think I would have the right to information.";

"It is important to recognise students with HIV while protecting others' right to information."

In brief, the commenters on Zhihu are convinced of the "incurable" nature of HIV, concerned about consequences of HIV infection due to "uncontrollable" factors, and faced with two contradictory choices whether to disclose the identity of PLWHA to protect non-PLWHA or to conceal their identity to protect themselves. All these have led to a heated debate on the disclosure of their identity. This may be the reason why most non-PLWHA have the same attitudes and behaviour.

7.3.3 Whether to Disclose Identity Has Consequences for Subject Construction

The author returned from a field survey (interviewing PLWHA aged approximately 50 in a society of acquaintances about the employment and marital status of their children who are not infected with HIV) and conducted preliminary interviews on the attitudes and behaviour of the general public towards PLWHA and the corresponding attitudes of PLWHA. The results were unexpected for the author.

Article 39 of the *Regulations on AIDS Prevention and Control* first issued by the State Council of China on January 18, 2006 stipulates that no entity or individual shall disclose the names, addresses, workplaces, portraits, medical history data and other information that can be used to deduce the specific identity of PLWHA and their family members without the consent of the individuals themselves or their guardians. Considered from the perspective of PLWHA, the regulations assume that once their identity is made public, it will cause social panic, greatly affect their survival and development, and harm efforts in HIV prevention and control.

Nevertheless, our assumption often falls far short of what is presented in real life. In a society of acquaintances, their identity can be easily revealed. When they are infected with HIV, it quickly becomes known to those around. In the interview, they unanimously agreed that the stigma against them still existed, but the people around changed from being initially resistant to tolerant, which is a big step forward. The main reason for the decline in rejection lies not only in the increasing knowledge about HIV but also in their attitudes, interpersonal skills and mental states in which they are presented to the public.

For example, a person surnamed Zhang told the author that when a child in the countryside got married and held a wedding reception, the infected person sat at a certain seat, and no one wanted to share the table with him. Or if he went late and there was an empty seat, others would indicate with their eyes or words that he was not welcome. Nevertheless, without low self-esteem, he actively interacted with everyone else in the village, took care of his crops well and earned a relatively high annual income. This positive attitude towards people earned him respect from others, and he was more self-conscious. No other infected people appeared in the village.

As a result, despite the concerns of those around, there is no longer obvious stigma and rejection.

In terms of interpersonal interaction, the stigma and rejection of PLWHA by the general public has diminished, but there is still clear stigma and rejection in regard to the marriage of their children from the accounts of a few infected people interviewed. Non-infected people would not allow their children to marry those of infected people if they know that both or one of the parents is infected with HIV. As a result, most children of the infected people have difficulty marrying. Some of them would find a suitable match when going out to work and remarry because the health status of their parents is not known due to the long distance.

In rural areas, most of the infected people are from poor families. Once infected, they always turn to society for more support and will implicitly inform that they have a sick family member that needs the government and village committee to favour them with subsidies. In a society of acquaintances, people involved will endeavour to determine what kind of disease it is. In addition, there is a weak enforcement of the law in rural areas (the regulation that information about infected people must not be disclosed). Thus, information about them is made public in secret within a certain time and scope. However, there is no such social phenomenon as serious stigma if their identities are made public as we construct.

7.3.4 Possibility and Value of Disclosure of Identity

From a medical viewpoint, the country's free treatment for PLWHA aims to control the reproduction of HIV in their body and keep the viral load of HIV very low. HIV cannot be exterminated because it can be latent in the body's immune cells, and drugs can only kill HIV free in body fluids (blood, lymphatic fluid, semen, etc.). This creates a balance where the drugs cannot completely kill all HIV viruses, but the HIV viruses cannot continue to multiply to attack other immune cells in the body.

AIDS cannot be cured, but HIV is prevented from continuing to destroy the body's immune system, and people with high-risk behaviours are much more likely to be voluntarily monitored for timely treatment. Therefore, PLWHA can work and live normally to contribute to society rather than rely entirely on the government or add to the burden of other taxpayers.

Article 38 of the *Regulations on AIDS Prevention and Control* first issued by the State Council of China on January 18, 2006 stipulates that PLWHA have the obligation to inform their sexual partners of the fact of their infection or illness in a timely manner and truthfully inform their doctors of the fact of their infection or illness when they seek medical treatment. This aims to prevent the transmission of HIV to others. There are two consequences of informing sexual partners. First, their relationship will end if the partner is not infected after testing; second, their relationship may continue by depending on each other for survival, or the partner may appeal to law. Not all doctors will continue to treat them as other patients, and some, if not a few, will simply refuse or find excuses not to continue treating them.

In other words, disclosure of their identity to their sexual partners and doctors brings stigma and exclusion to them. Why not disclose their identity to the general public as stigma is inevitable?

The stigma and rejection of PLWHA ultimately results from the self-constructed risk of transmission and threat of death. When neither exists, disclosure becomes possible. When non-infected people are informed of the identity of those infected, they will protect themselves in their daily interactions and work. The risk of HIV transmission will thus be greatly reduced, which is a good thing for the public and the country. As individuals with initiative, PLWHA would make efforts to reduce rejection by others even if their identity should be disclosed.

7.3.5 Disclosure of Identity: Who, to Whom and How

For PLWHA, the daily experience of rejection has led to their subjective perception of an unsafe future and an extreme fear of people and things to which they are exposed. With medical treatment advances and media campaigns by the government and its relevant authorities, the stigma has changed from extreme fear to rational and tolerant treatment since the first case of HIV infection in China, but the stigma of being "marginalized" still remains. We cannot deny their initiative, although they continue to face stigma and exclusion in some areas. They may voluntarily inform others of their identity and gain the recognition and respect of others through positive attitudes towards work and life, thereby changing their stereotypes in the eyes of others and ultimately resolving conflict with others to reduce stigma and rejection.

For the general public, the level of knowledge about HIV does not completely eliminate the fear of contracting the virus. Most people believe when they are exposed to someone with HIV, they first develop a fear of the "dishonourable" route of infection (most believe HIV infection is predominantly attributed to sexual misconduct) and the misconception that if they become infected, they will die. Then, they voluntarily create a psychological barrier and subtly express a reluctance to expose themselves to the infected people, even with repulsive language and actions. They are constructed by the public based on their personal experience and speculation about the experience of others. In fact, if we are exposed to an infected person, the case might be different. In the era of highly developed medical disciplines, people's attitudes change from non-acceptance to acceptance, but there is still stigma and rejection in some areas. For instance, they may work together, but they must never be vague about exposure in daily life, such as eating, bathing or drinking, nor will they have a romantic or even sexual relationship with an infected person.

While the author does not fully subscribe to the view that the protection of privacy should give way to the rights of life and health when it threatens the life and health of others, the uncertainties of vulnerability to HIV infection must be considered. The extent and degree of exposure to an infected person in everyday life must also be considered. For example, in addition to doctors who treat them, their sexual partners and spouses, as stipulated in the *Regulations on AIDS Prevention and Control*, should the identity of infected people be disclosed to their other relatives and the small group of people in which they live and work? Rights to life and health are the most fundamental human rights. Thus, people in close exposure to them have the right to know their identity. We cannot ignore the right of health of others while protecting their privacy.

PLWHA show fear and anxiety about the world around because of their identity and will consciously keep a distance from others, a behaviour easily perceived by others. As mentioned earlier, in a community of acquaintances, information about them is quickly made known. If they conceal their identity in advance out of good will or for various reasons, they will be thrown into an unfavorable situation once revealed and will be labelled as "immoral" or "insincere", which will result in increased fear and more serious stigma and rejection. Thus, we suggest that they voluntarily disclose their identity ahead of everyone else to address stigma and change from being those who need to manage information to being those who need to handle an embarrassing social situation. It is believed that they will think things over before voluntarily disclosing their identity and adopt corresponding strategies to deal with the possible consequences after disclosure.

Reference

Global health sector strategy on HIV: 2016–2021 Towards ending AIDS [EB/OL]. https://apps.who.int/iris/bitstream/handle/10665/246178/WHO-HIV-2016.05-eng.pdf?sequence=1

Chapter 8
Research Findings and Prospects

8.1 Research Findings

8.1.1 Research Conclusions

8.1.1.1 The Formation of Stigma Against People Living with HIV/AIDS is a Complex and Multi-Faceted Process

PLWHA experience stigma and discrimination in the mental, working, medical care, schooling and other areas. The study found that stigma manifests itself in moral degradation, employment discrimination, refusal of doctors to treat or indifferent treatment, isolation and rejection of students living with HIV/AIDS by schools, teachers and peer groups, and a complex and diverse range of discriminatory behaviours in these areas respectively.

The mechanisms of stigmatisation of PLWHA in China are the result of the intertwined and combined effects between the individual, group and social levels.

The individual-level mechanism of stigmatisation of PLWHA is based on attribution theory from the social psychology perspective, which centers on "controllability". This means that the causes of HIV infection are divided into controllable and uncontrollable aspects. If the cause of infection is considered to be controllable, stigma and discrimination are usually attached to the infection, such as through sexual misconduct and drug abuse. Conversely, the uncontrollable attribution brings sympathy to them, such as babies infected through blood transfusion or mother-to-child transmission, who will gain more sympathy from the public.

The group-level stigmatisation of PLWHA is a self-protective and psychological defence mechanism for the social group. The public stigmatises them because of the threat they feel from the AIDS community and fear of the high infectivity of the disease. They exclude PLWHA from their own sphere of life or group for self-protection. Thus, the group-level mechanism elevates stigma to a moral level.

The social-level mechanism of stigmatisation of PLWHA is based on social morality theory. The understanding of the mechanisms of stigma and discrimination

X. Wang, *Destigmatisation of People Living with HIV/AIDS in China*, A Sociological View of AIDS, https://doi.org/10.1007/978-981-16-8534-7_8

should not be limited to the individual and group levels but should be a sociocultural phenomenon linked to the human community as a whole. Stigma is not an isolated social phenomenon but is closely related to culture, power and difference. Ultimately, the formation of stigma is linked to inequalities in social structures. PLWHA are generally subject to social exclusion and discrimination, and most of the infections are associated with their low socio-economic status, poverty and unfortunate life experiences. They are stigmatised and discriminated against for engaging in high-risk activities. After infection, they are further stigmatised and deprived of more social resources, creating a vicious cycle of inequality.

The stigma against them has been associated with the key targets of HIV prevention and control in China since its inception, such as clandestine prostitutes, male homosexuals, injecting drug users and paid blood sellers.

8.1.1.2 Evolving Features of and New Changes in HIV Stigma Based on Symbolic and Instrumental Stigmas

HIV stigma includes symbolic stigma based on concepts and instrumental stigma characterised by symptoms of the disease. The evolution of symbolic stigma can be presented based on the concept of AIDS. The conceptual name of AIDS in China has changed from politically stigmatised "aizibing" (爱资病), to sexually stigmatised "aizibing" (爱滋病), which condemns sexual misconduct, and to value-neutral destigmatised "aizibing" (艾滋病). A conceptual or symbolic destigmatisation of AIDS has been basically achieved in China.

Instrumental stigma refers to the fear resulting from a lack of adequate information about the symptoms and transmission modes of AIDS. It has evolved from scary physical symptoms to manageable physical manifestations in HIV prevention strategies, from incurability to manageability in medical treatments, from physical contacts to fixed modes of transmission in transmission modes, from "sexual-only" transmission to multiple modes of infection in infection modes, and from "blame-oneself-only theory" to "innocence theory" in the basic argument.

The symbolic stigma and instrumental stigma form an interactive evolutionary process, with the former providing the basis or tone for the latter and the latter further developing the stigma on the basis of the former.

There are new changes in the stigmatisation of PLWHA: the stigma therein is still prevalent in society, and there is a shift from the predominantly symbolic stigma to the predominantly instrumental stigma. However, the mutual stigma between PLWHA and the high-risk population makes the more insidious forms of stigma spread from the public to individuals.

8.1.1.3 Negative Impact of HIV Stigma on People Living with HIV/AIDS and Society

Stigma affects PLWHA at the individual, group and social levels.

At the individual level, firstly, stigma causes chronic fear, depression and, in many cases, suicidal tendency and revenge mentality among them. Secondly, it causes them to conceal their illness from their family and friends, which could have more serious consequences. Thirdly, it leads to the destruction of social networks and loss of social capital, which could lead to further internalisation of stigma and self-loathing. At the group level, the impact is shown in the stigma against their family members and destruction of family relationships. At the social level, it undermines social justice, stability and unity, weakens social integration, and even damages the image of the government.

As shown in previous studies, the emotions of PLWHA often result from a mixture of stress, distress and frustration experienced by people concerned or their personality factors and are considered one of the important indicators. However, the subjects in this study had less pronounced or very mild mood swings and were generally not very different from the past, although with some signs of depression.

If PLWHA show stronger negative emotions in areas such as help, self-stigma, social stigma and hiding their illness, they tend to think that seeking help is something to be ashamed of in that they would be rejected by others and their self-confidence and sense of self-worth would be diminished. They also tend to keep their secrets. As a result, they are more emotionally unstable and less likely to seek help.

In addition, they have a very complex and unstable psychological state in the early stages. They want to solve problems on their own, but they have to wait because of some limitations. Thus, the degree of self-stigma is consistent with delay in seeking help, which is more evident among women infected with HIV.

Some studies hold that interviewees are often unable to avoid the threat of stigma. Although the effects of stigma have been partially weakened during their training in counselling, they still have to overcome stigma and helplessness before actually seeking help. Some of them stress that they will never seek help until the last minute. For most infected people, revealing their plight and privacy in front of others is not only embarrassing but also makes them feel helpless, which is one of the reasons why many of them would rather continue to suffer than seek help.

This study does not differ significantly from previous studies in terms of social stigma and shows that when PLWHA are aware that they are discriminated against, they experience feelings of social rejection and are more likely to feel deprived of various resources and face unequal distribution of social resources.

Evaluation of negative ego personality can also cause individuals to develop a sense of stigma from public relations. Evaluation of ego personality represents an assessment of interpersonal interactions and social competence. When people perceive themselves as positive, trustworthy and useful, they have a higher self-evaluation rating and are more likely to believe they have sufficient ability, resources and action to achieve their goals when faced with stress and adversity. Conversely, when people think themselves as a failure or something, they naturally do not have the ability to deal with problems positively and are prone to withdrawal, self-abandonment and a greater sense of stigma in their lives. Research has found that PLWHA tend to withdraw as a response to stigma, which in turn brings about limited life opportunities and leads to a vicious cycle of social support systems.

8.1.2 Related Discussions

8.1.2.1 Discussion of Stigma

Previous research has suggested that individuals comply with public opinions because they are influenced by social norms. The point is that individuals will change their behaviour to conform to the normative standards of the group to avoid violating the norms. The author argues that social stigma is concomitant with self-identity. It is possible for people to be influenced by social stigma and change their self-identity and to change themselves and recognise their identity before they are stigmatised. Thus, the relationship between self-labelling and public stigmatisation of infected people and alienation from intimate relationships, if proven, may need to be grounded in more contexts and more appropriately illustrated by other research tools or data.

Post-stigma emotions are a common feature of psychological distress or combined manifestations in the infected people and are one of the main motivating factors for their deviant behaviour. If stigma can be addressed early and professionally, it can not only prevent the deterioration of psychological symptoms but also maximise the efficacy of treatment. Many studies have shown that stigmatised emotions or psychological distortions are influenced by physiological, psychological and social factors. Thus, providing interventions such as counselling or psychotherapy is the long-recognised practice considered the most appropriate approach in early prevention and intervention. Those who receive counselling and treatment early are better able to establish themselves in a good living environment.

The study concludes that there is a correlation between infected people's emotions and help-seeking behaviour, which seems to be inconsistent with the findings of previous studies. Some scholars have suggested that high levels of stress, depression, family conflict and financial stress can predict whether a person will seek counselling. Others have suggested that there is no association between the level of psychological distress and attempts to seek help or help-seeking behaviour. In conclusion, the infected people's mood is an important factor in influencing their help-seeking behaviour, but its specific circumstances and operational mechanisms are not discussed in the study.

Stigma is also shown in avoidance behaviours (avoidance, hiding, secrecy, etc.), which has an important influence on help-seeking attitudes or behaviours. Self-stigma plays an important role in the emotions and avoidance behaviour of the infected people. The severer the stigma, the more likely they tend to avoid and not seek help.

8.1.2.2 Stigma and High-Risk Populations

In the author's view, one of the most important criteria for defining the "high-risk population" is the mode of transmission, but further analysis by tracing back the process of infection shows that the model of classifying people as "high-risk populations" is actually very limited. For instance, gay men belong to high-risk populations because anal sex may lead to microvascular rupture and increase the chance of infection. In fact, not all of them engage in condomless anal sex, and anal sex is not only a sexual practice restricted to gay men. Some researchers have thus preferred the concept of "risky behaviour" to that of "high-risk population".

Epidemiologists tend to define risk in terms of high-risk populations rather than risky behaviours because the former is categorised in a socially established way, which makes them easier to find. By defining the high-risk population, risk begins to be fixed within a seemingly specific population, who becomes visible and homogeneous, distinguishing it from others in transmission rates.

From a public health perspective, it is difficult to monitor or detect such a specific group of people. Among the author's interviewees, homosexuals are often reluctant to identify themselves because of social pressure and stigma. As a result, epidemiologists do not know where their subjects are when conducting research or are confused about how to distinguish or identify their homosexuality. This is a new way of classifying people in an attempt by epidemiologists to find true high-risk populations, trying to distinguish between identity and behaviour. As a result, any man who has sex with another man is included, whether he identifies himself as a gay, bisexual, heterosexual or other identity. However, this does not accurately convey the meaning of HIV risky behaviour and even extends the scope of risk to a wider range of people. Ultimately, this classification of high-risk populations is likely to have become a major source of stigma and discrimination.

8.1.3 Following Questions of the Study

Stigma, especially self-stigma, is difficult to reduce or alleviate by means of publicity and education. The author found in his study that the self-stigma of PLWHA was reduced after mutual understanding was established at a counselling occasion. Although this finding cannot exclude the influence of social expectations, it is at least another consideration to reduce the impact of stigma. This is because they most need help and are most likely to receive treatment after counselling. If the stigma of this group of people can be reduced through means such as education or less threatening counselling, the likelihood of addressing their distress through counselling and consultation increases.

The author witnessed the case of a doctor wearing gloves to test the blood of a person infected with HIV and then wiping the table with alcohol. Why are doctors who are relatively well protected still so fearful of AIDS? Exposed to a dangerous infectious disease, the doctor cleaned his surroundings to re-establish a clean environment, which was utter stigma and discrimination for the infected person.

Previous sources have shown that the disease in modern political discourse is often metaphorically used in the era of Western totalitarianism. Thus, the "disease" is not just a physiological issue but something that symbolises evil and has to be punished.

This means that the stereotype of AIDS has a deep sociocultural context. How does AIDS evolve from a "personal disease" to a "cultural disease"? Let us look at the disease from a cultural perspective and examine the correlation between stigma and AIDS and the hidden social meaning of stigma.

Previous research found that along with systematic classification, social order is then introduced to delineate the symbolic boundaries of things, objects, and activities. This boundary illustrates the actual placement and moral beliefs. The more powerful groups in society accordingly assign negative stereotypes to others, whose rights, cultures or languages are long ignored by society. Based on previous research findings, the author found that the stigmatised others internalised the moral and value indoctrination of the dominant society after a long period of discipline by the dominant culture and thus became self-stigmatised.

Erving Goffman argued that attributes of some stigmas, such as physical appearance, disfigurement or skin colour, are not readily visible, for instance, in PLWHA and psychiatric patients. Thus, in contrast to the readily visible explicit stigmas (such as obesity), these implicit stigmas can go undetected through information control and covering (Goffman 1963). In terms of stigma classification, being infected with HIV from condomless sex is seen as a disgusting physical or unhealthy defect. Sex itself is interspersed with ideologies of sexual morality and reproduction-oriented sex, creating a double stigma for those infected through sex. One of the interviewees, a civil service administrator, also believed that having AIDS is self-inflicted and will lead to an embarrassing and ugly death, except for those unfortunate enough to be forced into infection. Homosexuality, prostitution, promiscuity and drug abuse are labelled bad. Once stigmatised as such, the infected people are treated differently and even ostracised by members of the group to which they belong.

In addition to the stigma of the disease, PLWHA have stigmas such as homosexuality, drug abuse and sex trafficking. The frustration caused by HIV infection can also have a significant impact on their outlook on life. It often takes time to re-examine the value of their existence and readjust themselves. This study also found that they face a variety of physical and mental problems, such as social exclusion, social fear, and physical and mental fatigue. HIV infection may also be accompanied by discriminatory attitudes, resulting in depression and social isolation. This is their self-protection to maintain a moderate distance from the outside world.

In the interviews with them, which attempted to use stigma as a point of inquiry, the author felt that they were vulnerable people in real need of help. The words "intervention", "prevention and treatment" and "correction" appear frequently in various sources and academic journals, but there is a lack of research on their needs. This may put these researchers on the same footing as the general public and may have unwittingly had different forms of tendentious discriminatory attitudes and behaviours. Before the improvement of the overall context, it will be difficult to reduce discrimination and stigma against them among the general public.

Furthermore, in the process of studying help-seeking, this study extends its research theme from the help-seeking attitude to the help-seeking behaviour and explores whether the latter is one of the important elements influencing the former. Apart from exploring more directly the help-seeking behaviour that is of most concern to researchers and practitioners, the findings of the study can serve as a basis for following researchers to discuss help-seeking behaviour.

8.1.4 Research Limitations

8.1.4.1 Limitations

The results of this study reflect the emphasis on the understanding of problems rather than the representativeness of the population by aid agencies, mental health-related agencies and higher education institutions. The interviewees selected included PLWHA, people and things they may come into contact with and those they would turn to when in need. The author did not take a quantitative approach to the analysis but tried to be objective and neutral. Nonetheless, some staff or the infected people were not willing to be interviewed because of privacy concerns, somewhat affecting the conclusions of the study.

In the early stages of contact with the infected people, the author had some established preconceptions in heterosexuality, for instance, that the one-for-one relationship is taken for granted; that it is only acceptable to have a courtship before having sex; or that it is unacceptable if they continue to visit obscene places for sex even after their infection. These thoughts made it difficult for the author to understand what the interviewees said and even made him misunderstand them. It was only through repeated reading of the materials, reflecting on the questions raised in the interviews and discussing with scholars various social contexts of PLWHA and homosexuals that the author gradually revised his understanding and no longer interpreted the phenomenon using established concepts.

As a male researcher, the author discussed the issue of sexuality and stigma with male homosexuals. They said that they could discuss it more freely without worrying about transferring their feelings or disclosure of their identity since the objects of their desire were men and the author was not a member of the homosexual community. One point to mention here is that, as the author had no experience of living with PLWHA, he was initially uncomfortable in contact with them for fear that his behaviour and demeanour would reveal rejection or fear, possibly confirming the labelling behaviour towards them. Thus, he was cautious in every way, which made the interviewees nervous and the interview situation relatively less safe and comfortable and may affect their expression. After several contacts, the author experienced their sincerity and willingness to share and understood that they were not free to express whatever they wanted to. The previous tension was actually a projection of the author's inner self onto them. Then, after overcoming his anxiety, the author could face the interview situation more comfortably and gradually forget the presence of the AIDS marker.

The study respected the wishes of the interviewees, who had the right to decide whether to be interviewed and to return a visit. There were fewer refusals in the study, but the refusal rate was higher when home visits were conducted because some of them would consider the feelings of their family members. Thus, the level of literacy among those who were willing to participate in the interview was relatively higher among staff and relatively lower among PLWHA. Some case interviews were terminated for specific reasons. In addition, those who denied or could not detect whether they suffered from stigma may have underestimated their level of awareness, which was one of the limitations of this study.

8.1.4.2 Reflections

In the process of conceptualising the research framework, the author encountered many difficulties. Firstly, PLWHA belong to a very complex group. It is a complicated and intricate thing in terms of the concept of stigma and demand behaviour. How does the author study stigma labels and demand behaviour? How should we view other different service methods? Where do other different forms of help fit into the hierarchy of help-seeking? These are the questions that the author has to face.

The choice of approaches to study stigma is something that a researcher needs to consider. At first, the author thought that counselling was the only and best option, but he slowly shifted from a self-centred to a respondent-centred perspective as the direction of the research was established. In fact, there are many interpretations of stigma in the broad sense, but only the interviewees have the right to decide what kind of stigma it is. As a researcher, the author chooses to explore ways to remove stigma using counselling and wishes to include the elements that have been identified in the research. It is not the focus of this study to discuss how the interviewees choose other means of help or whether they have sought other means of help before receiving counselling.

Social stigma is present at all levels of society, but deeply rooted social networks are still deeply embedded in blood relations. In exploring the elements of stigma for PLWHA, it is important to consider the influence of age group, education, work experience and the size of interpersonal networks and that of gender, differences of special groups, and marital status. We look forward to further relevant research on the specific criteria of stigma that can be experienced by the infected people in real life.

Secondly, it is important to return to the inner world of the infected people. As they go through the shock of the diagnosis of the disease and the initial panic of the unknown, they gradually resume a normal life and have a growing need for intimacy. Some people choose to give up and stop pursuing love, shifting the focus of their lives, but many others are torn between wanting to love and not daring to, as well as between wanting to have sex and being afraid of transmitting the virus.

The words of the interviewees in the study continue to haunt the author. They hold that although there are indeed many uncertainties in the emotional bonding of the gay community, they can try love and sex before infection because they are healthy. Nonetheless, after infection, their desire to pursue love and sex is limited by the society and themselves. Thus, they must first be liberated from the constraints of social morality if they want to find intimacy of their own. This is not a disorderly and out-of-control phenomenon but rather a discovery of what they expect from intimacy through groping. After this process of hesitation characterised by moving backwards in some cases and watching and waiting in other cases, the infected people gradually accept themselves, allow themselves to have intimacy of their own and even transform the relationship into a purely emotional encounter.

This process, however, does not move forward in one direction but goes back and forth. According to the different situations of the infected people, they may temporarily stay in a state of intimacy. It is a dynamic process, perhaps adjusted due to time, personal inner growth or change. In their stereotype, their love is always sad and unproductive, causing some to give up the expectation of finding true love and avoid being hurt by not being involved in affection. This is a form of self-protection for them in the pursuit of intimacy. Reducing expectations due to fear of loss is another adjustment that they make in facing intimacy. This may be mixed with the uncertainty of maintaining the intimacy as homosexual individuals, but the choice to reduce their emotional yearnings after infection and make themselves more comfortable in such relationships seems to have become irreversible helplessness and destiny.

Furthermore, the infected people often suffer from acute opportunistic infections that threaten their lives because AIDS is a syndrome. As a result, the mentality that some of them may become ill or die at any time has strengthened the feeling that the future is unpredictable. When they are looking forward to a relationship, the desire to try but the fear of failure often makes them feel like a toddler, not being able to take the first steady step towards intimacy. Even after the first step towards meeting someone, the fear of commitment and the uncertainty of the existence of a relationship as it develops is often a factor in their hesitation to move forward. Additionally, they fear that their feelings will be hurt and thus tend to hesitate. One interviewee spoke of how she was emotionally focused and impulsive whenever she was in a relationship, but was afraid of repeating the same mistakes she had made. Therefore, when the other person was willing to accept her, she did not want to be a burden to him for health reasons or to be taken care of in an unequal relationship, which prevented them from starting a new relationship.

Just as the emotional intimacy will "end" for them, the infected people have problems with sex. They are reserved about sex or hesitate to have sex, although they have tried to take protective measures. One married interviewee mentioned that his wife had said that she expected more sexual contact in addition to emotional companionship, even if she would be infected through sex. Rather than being encouraged by this from his intimate partner, he was made more reticent about sex because of the risk of infection. Such a passive mindset seemed to tell him that HIV infection was a given fact and that, if she chose to leave him because he was infected, it seemed that he had no right to change it. Faced with such a decision by his beloved wife, he did not know what to do. The author finds that among the hesitations and contradictions, the infected people will think over and over again, as if they believe that contracting the virus is a mistake that needs to be punished, so they have no right to choose and are not allowed to love others. However, as they move beyond the moral limits and get closer to what they truly want, they realise that they still need to have intimate relationships. Despite HIV infection, they do not allow past experience to hinder the development of their future intimate relationships.

8.2 Research Prospects

In the pluralistic society of the twenty-first century, there is the wanton imposition of stigma on PLWHA and the narrowing and deprivation of their space for survival. After understanding their feelings and listening to their deepest voices, the author attempts to explore the factors contributing to the formation of HIV stigma under the influence of multiple subjective and objective factors and to analyse the possibility for them to be discriminated against or victimised under the influence of stigma. The study aims to eliminate HIV stigma and discrimination against them, with the ultimate aim of preventing discrimination and inequality and giving them favourable space for survival.

8.2.1 Revision of AIDS Health Education

Firstly, the current health education campaigns focus on the safe sex of PLWHA. Some interviewees in the study mentioned that simply showing the dangers and threats of HIV or the importance of safe sex is not enough to motivate them to use condoms, details on how to do this should be provided, and ways such as caressing, touching or kissing can be used to increase sexual satisfaction.

Health education should be extended to the general public to make them understand what HIV is and know that the infected people are no different from non-infected people in that they have the same needs and expectations for intimacy and the right to love, intimacy and sex.

Although previous studies have suggested that the expectations and pursuits of emotional relationships among male homosexuals are similar to those of heterosexuals, it cannot be inferred that the partnership of heterosexuals infected with HIV will have the same change. As the proportion of heterosexuals is increasing and the intimacy is not exclusive to male homosexuals, a more comprehensive understanding of the infected people would be gained by contact with more heterosexual cases in the research.

In future research, if we compare the state of intimacy based on the length of infection, identify more clearly the temporal changes in intimacy, and compare them with the course of the disease, perhaps we can better predict the impact and difficulties of intimacy that the infected people may experience at different periods of time.

Secondly, when planning the information strategy of AIDS websites in the publicity and education via online counselling, the first thing to consider is to diversify the publicity items, increase the content of prevention capabilities, and adopt different appeal methods for different target groups to achieve greater effectiveness.

AIDS-related websites mainly provide information on basic medical knowledge, transmission routes, prevention methods, etc. There is a need to enrich the information on psychological counselling, daily life adjustment, exercise, diet and nutrition after the onset of the disease, and regulations on the protection of the basic rights and interests on the part of the infected people, the guiding principle for doctors to treat AIDS and the comprehensive protection of health care workers. On some foreign websites, there are various models for assessing AIDS-related issues and ways to help, which are mostly based on the number of indicators to determine the answers needed, but the use of quantitative scoring evaluation modes is still rare. As a result, there is a lack of consistent criteria for the websites of health education institutions to explore a range of related issues. For instance, there is no definitive answer as to how many categories are considered adequate.

According to some researchers, the authenticity of online information is one of the most criticised aspects characterised by uneven quality, lack of accuracy and a wide range of material. As members of the network join voluntarily and aim to collaborate and share resources with each other, the quality of the resources is not yet good and needs to be identified by users. The general public tends to place their trust in medical practitioners and the medicines, products or treatments recommended in medical information. Nevertheless, some websites often exaggerate the efficacy of their products or deliberately conceal their side effects for commercial benefits. At present, most of the audiences of AIDS websites are the general public and homosexuals, but different target groups have their own specific information needs, so the government's policy of subsidising private organisations to set up AIDS websites does need to be adjusted. Private groups should be encouraged to specify their target groups on websites to avoid duplication with others and provide tailored information to meet the needs of website users infected with HIV.

Health authorities for AIDS prevention and control should construct online virtual museums of AIDS and create information exchange channels such as an electronic newspaper, which should be directly linked to the AIDS websites of other countries. An information exchange platform could also be set up on a trial basis with neighbouring countries to effectively identify the infected people among the mobile population and to supplement each other's incomplete information, which could provide a more convenient search method for those who need it. Of course, websites should effectively label all sources of information and explain specific terms.

The information on AIDS websites in China is relatively poor and needs to be enriched. In the author's view, a special communication forum should be created on the websites of government departments to open discussion space to enhance interaction with users, provide timely psychological counselling and answer their questions about AIDS. The health authorities can encourage such organisations to adopt self-regulatory measures through financial subsidies or counselling and educate users on how to recognise the correctness and reliability of websites to avoid deception and consequent damage to health.

8.2.2 *Innovations in Social Services for People Living with HIV/AIDS*

8.2.2.1 Linkage of HIV Services with Social Welfare

The study found that the AIDS service system is not yet linked to social welfare, and the departments to which it belongs are not very clear. Additionally, it is well separated from the police system. For instance, when PLWHA commit crimes, the police often do not know what to do when they arrive because they are afraid of taking over the case because of the special identity. In many countries, AIDS-related social workers have taken on a vital role in the advocacy of rights, service delivery and promotion of diverse social functions, including dialogue with the government, community engagement, advocacy of rights and client support. However, there is a tendency for government social welfare entities and non-AIDS departments to refer the infected people to specialised service organisations. The common service targets of the community where they are located include street vagrants, people with disabilities, people who commit domestic violence, people with mental disorders, and the elderly. In regard to the infected people, the community is concerned only with the identity of the disease. It has been a long-standing problem to link HIV services with the social welfare system. Civil affairs departments have also directly shown that there is nothing they can do to settle them. However, some social workers in the interviews were enthusiastic in their attempts to link AIDS with social welfare through constant phone calls, door-to-door applications, cross-sectoral presentations and participation in societies.

The author observes that social welfare agencies still devote few resources to the care of PLWHA and thinks that this does not seem to help. AIDS has always been regarded as a chronic disease with specific transmission routes. The infected people do not require long-term medical care or special treatment, and most of them without symptoms return to the community to live with their family and friends. Some of them have good community support systems, so those without special needs may not get in contact with community agencies for the rest of their lives. Nonetheless, some of them who have concealed their illness to those around may seek support from community services or peers in the community or may urgently seek eligible community agencies. For instance, those who need resettlement may seek shelter, and those whose rights have been compromised and need to lodge a complaint may turn to rights promotion agencies.

8.2.2.2 Institutional Treatment Services

The provision of clinical support services or mutual support for PLWHA is appropriate and necessary. Although at the initial stage of this study the institutional model might affect the attitudes of some of them due to unfamiliarity, the author found from several interviewees that if the institution provided a safe and comfortable space for them to express, discuss and share their experiences with each other, the unfamiliarity would be eliminated. In particular, those wardmates were able to support each other through mutual recognition.

Group interaction with the help of professionals can reproduce the interaction pattern of intimate partners of the infected people and apply it to real-life situations. If they have specific adjustment problems, for example, if they do not know how to communicate with their intimate partners, short-term targeted counselling can be provided to help them solve the problem and develop a problem-solving model of their own. For those with long-term adjustment problems, such as HIV-related affective disorders, long-term targeted counselling may be provided as appropriate. For those whose intimate relationship has been affected by the infection, targeted therapies can be used to improve understanding of the disease and self-acceptance, aiming at a return to the partnership. The ability to express themselves and the ability to deal with the disease should be improved. They and their partners can receive individual or group treatments, identify patterns of interaction with each other and modify or establish new interactions through the assistance of the therapist.

8.2.3 Improved Conditions for Social Survival of People Living with HIV/AIDS

8.2.3.1 Safeguarding Basic Rights and Interests

The most important thing the government health departments need to do is to uphold administrative fairness, act in accordance with the law and set a good example for special groups. To give a simple example, students and teachers in primary schools for the AIDS population should be entitled to the same social benefits as ordinary children and workers and should not be denied their entitlements because they have already received some of the benefits. If government departments do not provide corresponding benefits to them, how should they provide the benefits, especially basic human rights, to the disadvantaged groups in society? When AIDS turns from a terminal disease to a chronic one, the infected people are only required to receive treatment, or HIV prevention campaigns are only conducted for the public under previous health policies, which has been ineffective in controlling the epidemic. There have been numerous incidents of rights violations of the infected people, which have caused much controversy. Thus, the protection of their human rights should be on the agenda.

Although some free medical resources for the infected people are available and some human rights protection policies are introduced in the current policies in China, those policies have not been fully implemented. The author observed several incidents in which shop assistants asked the infected people to leave immediately after their identities had been revealed in public places. After their self-stigma and social stigma were established, they did not complain, but chose to leave in silence for fear that more people around them would learn of their special identity. The managers of the services also hold that the corresponding policies have not truly been implemented. Most of the infected people are concerned about their privacy. Even if there is a policy in place, few of them will actually file a complaint if their rights are compromised. Thus, there is an urgent need to put protection regulations into practice.

8.2.3.2 Promotion of Diversified Education

HIV stigma is mostly due to negative stereotypes and prejudices. Thus, to reduce discrimination and stigma against the infected people, we must first change such stereotypes and prejudices, which truly needs the help of diversified education to improve their living environment. The school education system can help students understand the value of multiculturalism, such as the gender subject, origin of the disease and characteristics, teach them how to respect differences and accept the diversity of special groups, and guide them to discard old ideas, a tendency to discriminate, prejudice and stereotypes in an ultimate effort to develop their newer and more diverse mindsets.

In this study, the author found that he and several health care workers interviewed were not familiar with how to understand the intimate relationships of the infected people. Thus, when caring for them or assisting them in dealing with intimate relationships, health care workers can first prepare themselves by reading books or accessing relevant information to increase their familiarity with this group, detecting inappropriate emotions in the interviews for correction, increasing their sensitivity to the issue of intimate relationships, and using feedback from the infected people to constantly modify their attitudes during the interaction.

8.2.3.3 Preventing the Spread of HIV

According to relevant sources, the number of PLWHA increases year by year in China, which has become a problem that urgently needs to be solved. The equation of the infected population with insecurity is the biggest obstacle to eliminating stigma and has had serious consequences, making them live in a more hidden way and posing greater difficulties for the elimination of HIV stigma and the overall HIV prevention and treatment.

It is all the more important for government authorities to integrate relevant departments such as education, health, civil affairs and public security, adopt a cross-sectoral approach to cooperation, and convey to the public the message that the HIV prevention and treatment project must be developed forever. This will be more effective in preventing the continued increase in the number of the infected people.

Firstly, AIDS-related rights protection and counselling agencies should be set up, and specialised agencies should be set up in government organisations at all levels in line with the mechanisms for vagrant sheltering, juvenile delinquency sheltering and domestic violence prevention and control. Secondly, the existing private counselling agencies should be integrated to provide counselling assistance and care for PLWHA in their families, schools, workplaces, mental health and personal emotions. In particular, support should be given to them in electing their representatives to seek legal assistance in accordance with relevant laws and regulations to truly implement the government's established policies of caring for the disadvantaged groups.

Reference

Goffman E (1963) Stigma: notes on the management of spoiled identity. Prentice-Hall, Inc.

Appendix A

Information of the Interviewees

No	Name	Sex	Age	Education	Status of infection	Occupation	Number of interviewed
1	ZHY	Male	43	Postgraduate	Non-infected	Director of the Office of the Civil Affairs Bureau	2
2	WSH	Male	Not clear	Postgraduate	Non-infected	Division Chief of the Office of the Civil Affairs Bureau	1
3	FUK	Male	53	Postgraduate	Non-infected	Staff of the Office of the Civil Affairs Bureau	2
4	WD	Female	42	University	Non-infected	Director of some institution	3
5	YTF	Female	34	University	Non-infected	Section chief of some institution	7
6	LG	Female	25	Postgraduate	Non-infected	Social worker	7
7	ZGY	Female	54	Not clear	Non-infected	Teacher	7
8	CR	Male	47	University	Non-infected	Staff of some institution	3
9	QDT	Male	63	Not clear	Non-infected	Social worker	8

(continued)

X. Wang, *Destigmatisation of People Living with HIV/AIDS in China*, A Sociological View of AIDS, https://doi.org/10.1007/978-981-16-8534-7

(continued)

No	Name	Sex	Age	Education	Status of infection	Occupation	Number of interviewed
10	KY	Male	28	University	Infected	Worker	7
11	FTY	Male	52	Junior middle school	Infected	Worker	6
12	ZFR	Female	37	Junior middle school	Infected	Unemployment	12
13	BU	Female	21	Junior middle school	Infected	Part-time job	5
14	NGT	Female	38	University	Infected	Unemployment	6
15	KUH	Female	24	Postgraduate	Infected	Unemployment	8
16	CDE	Male	34	Postgraduate	Infected	Unemployment	4
17	KUH	Female	32	University	Infected	Unemployment	2
18	HU	Female	46	Junior college	Infected	Unemployment	2
19	KI	Male	54	Graduate	Infected	Unemployment	7
20	DE	Female	30	Junior college	Infected	Unemployment	9
21	SEY	Male	37	Junior middle school	Infected	Enterprise	6
22	GRD	Male	25	Junior college	Infected	Unemployment	7
23	LI	Female	45	University	Infected	Part-time job	4
24	WA	Male	28	Polytechnic school	Infected	Unemployment	3
25	FUJ	Female	23	Junior college	Infected	Unemployment	3
26	LCL	Male	18	University	Infected	Student	4
27	ZZY	Male	19	University	Infected	Student	4
28	GQ	Male	20	University	Infected	Student	5
29	CHH	Female	20	University	Infected	Student	3
30	ZLX	Male	25	High school	Infected	Unemployment	4
31	XL	Female	36	High school	Infected	Part-time job	2
32	GQ	Male	32	University	Infected	Worker	3
33	WWZ	Male	26	Polytechnic school	Infected	Unemployment	6
34	LJJ	Male	21	University	Infected	Unemployment	4
35	LL	Male	44	Junior middle school	Infected	Unemployment	6
36	MXW	Female	30	University	Infected	Unemployment	4
37	ZLR	Male	15	Junior middle school	Infected	Student	5
38	CHL	Male	19	University	Infected	Student	5
39	GTD	Male	22	Postgraduate	Infected	Part-time job	3
40	MHL	Male	31	Postgraduate	Non-infected	Part-time job	7
41	DSE	Male	35	University	Non-infected	Part-time job	6

(continued)

(continued)

No	Name	Sex	Age	Education	Status of infection	Occupation	Number of interviewed
42	CS	Male	42	High school	Non-infected	Part-time job	8
43	MH	Male	26	University	Non-infected	Enterprise	2
44	LT	Female	23	Junior college	Non-infected	Student	9
45	CDU	Male	32	High school	Non-infected	Part-time job	5
46	LJK	Female	32	University	Non-infected	Enterprise	2
47	FAF	Male	25	University	Non-infected	Enterprise	4
48	MDF	Female	37	University	Non-infected	Medical Staff	6

Notes

To strictly adhere to academic ethics and protect the privacy of the interviewees, all the above names are replaced by the initials of their names. The author conducted several interviews at civil affairs departments, social work agencies, and "Red Ribbon" schools through meetings and online chats to obtain more materials.

The managers and workers of these agencies mainly described the functions of the agencies and the situations they were facing, including their work experiences. Some of the interviewees did not go into detail but mainly stated policies, which was still very helpful to the research.

Some of the interviews were conducted between the author and one interviewee, while others were conducted in groups of two or three, and some of the infected persons were interviewed accompanied by professional social workers or agency staff occasionally.

The author started to pay attention to PLWHA during college, and the paper for master's degree centred on the topic. Many interview data and personal experiences between 2004 and 2010 laid a good research foundation for the completion of doctoral theses and provided much information and facilities for finding the interviewees.

The study spanned the period from spring 2011 to early 2015, and 48 interviewees were interviewed and followed up several times. The interviewees were mainly from cities of Shanxi Province, as well as Beijing, Kunming, and some cities of Hebei Province. Most of the interview sites were chosen in parks, restaurants, institutions, schools, squares, etc.

The non-infected interviewees involved in the book are mainly a secondary reference between public and private spaces and between stigmatisation and destigmatisation and are particularly significant. The reason for this is that stigmatisation is not limited to infected people but also lies in the collateral relationship of the non-infected people. Therefore, it would be insufficient to study only infected individuals without interviewing non-infected individuals. Therefore, the non-infected people were involved in the study.

Appendix B

Outline of the Interview

1. **Interviews with PLWHA**

    (1) Name, age, education
    (2) Place of birth, household registration, time of entry
    (3) Family members, friends, contact status
    (4) Social adjustment, life troubles
    (5) What do you want to do now?
    (6) What did you do before you got sick? How about the income?
    (7) How did you get the disease?
    (8) How about the changes since you got sick?
    (9) What needs do you have now and can they be met?
    (10) Where have you been since you got sick?
    (11) Do you understand what people around you say about you?
    (12) What do your relatives and friends often say to you?
    (13) Do you know your health condition?
    (14) If you communicate with strangers, is there any barrier?
    (15) Do you know people around you who have the same disease?
    (16) How is life different from before?
    (17) Are there any difficulties in financial income and expenses now?
    (18) Are you satisfied with yourself now?
    (19) Have you received any psychological counselling?
    (20) What are the usual activities and ways to spend time?
    (21) Do you feel that you have a sense of existence?
    (22) Are there many people who help you?
    (23) Do you still have regular contact with your former acquaintances?
    (24) What are your own requirements?

2. Interviews with Relevant Staff

    (1) How much do you know about the group PLWHA?

X. Wang, *Destigmatisation of People Living with HIV/AIDS in China*, A Sociological View of AIDS, https://doi.org/10.1007/978-981-16-8534-7

(2) Are there many civil affairs staff who have received special training?
(3) Are they the target of social work help?
(4) How about the scope and objectives of support?
(5) Is there enough staff?
(6) What is the nature of the supporting organisations?
(7) Who guides them to the supporting organisations?
(8) Will they receive special help here?
(9) What if they don't receive help?
(10) Are they free here?
(11) When is the peak period of their infection being found?
(12) What is the biggest difficulty in helping?
(13) What will happen to them in the future?
(14) Can they get special rescue in case of illness?
(15) How do people in the community regard them?
(16) Can psychological counselling and assessment agencies help them?
(17) Will their family members be discriminated against?
(18) Can they be provided with specialized social assistance?
(19) Are they allowed to receive education or re-employment?

The manufacturer's authorised representative in the EU is Springer Nature Customer Service Centre GmbH, Europaplatz 3, 69115 Heidelberg, Germany. If you have any concerns regarding our products, please contact ProductSafety@springernature.com

Printed and bound by CPI Group (UK) Ltd, Croydon, CR0 4YY
30/09/2026
02225264-0009